# Nursing Studies Theory and Practice

**Ingrid Condell**

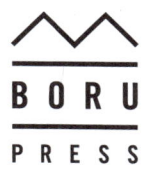

BORU PRESS

Boru Press Ltd.
The Farmyard
Birdhill
Co. Tipperary
www.borupress.ie

© Ingrid Condell 2021
Chapters 5 and 6 © Laura Pratt, DML Training 2021

ISBN 978 1 83841 3415
Design by Sarah McCoy
Print origination by Carole Lynch
Illustrations by Andriy Yankovskyy
Printed by GraphyCems Ltd, Spain

The paper used in this book is made from wood pulp
of managed forests. For every tree felled, at least one tree is planted,
thereby renewing natural resources.

All rights reserved. No part of this publication may be copied, reproduced
or transmitted in any form or by any means without written permission of
the publisher or else under the terms of any licence permitting limited
copyright issued by the Irish Copyright Licensing Agency.

A CIP catalogue record for this book is available from the British Library.

For permission to reproduce photographs and artworks, the author and
publisher gratefully acknowledge the following:

© Alamy 2, 5 © Department of Health 24 © Homecare Medical Supplies 116
© HSE 2, 25, 117 © iStock 26, 30, 107, 108, 109, 110, 115, 116, 121, 125 ©
Ingrid Condell 10, 16, 29, 116, 154, 165, 186 © INMO 13 © Laura Durcan
106 © Laura Pratt 93, 94, 95, 96, 97, 98, 99, 100, 101, 102, 103 © National
Screening Service 19 © NMBI 2, 19, 173, 174 © Rolling News 15 ©
Shutterstock 2, 3, 9, 108, 133, 134, 135, 150, 160, 180, 181, 182 © World
Health Organisation 113, 114

The author and publisher have made every effort to trace all copyright
holders, but if any has been inadvertently overlooked we would be pleased
to make the necessary arrangement at the first opportunity.

# Acknowledgments

This book was written at a time when the world was experiencing a pandemic. Throughout this period nurses have demonstrated their commitment to provide care to people in the most testing and challenging of circumstances. Nurses across the globe have displayed courage, resilience and adaptability and I would like to acknowledge this.

I would also like to pay tribute to the fourteen young girls who started their nursing journey with me in 1985, who grew and developed to become professional, experienced nurses, nurse managers, advance nurse practitioners, educators and nurse leaders.

Nursing requires a complex range of skills and intelligences: the cognitive ability to understand scientific principles, the ability to apply those principles in a physically skilful way and the emotional intelligence to do so with care and compassion.

Nursing is a science and an art.

> This book is dedicated to Ethel Bigley in Room 21,
> for her ability to find fun in everything.

# ABOUT THE AUTHORS

**Ingrid Condell BSc Nursing (Hons) MSc (Research)**

Ingrid Condell qualified as a Registered General Nurse in 1989, having trained in the Adelaide Hospital, Dublin. She was conferred with a BSc in Nursing from Athlone Institute of Technology in 2008 and an MSc by Research in 2011. Her research explored the knowledge and experiences of the first cohort of Nurse Prescribers in Ireland. Her work was subsequently published in the academic journal *Nurse Prescribing* in 2014.

Ingrid has over ten years' experience in Higher and Further Education sectors; as a lecturer at the Institute of Technology Carlow and as a tutor with Tipperary Education and Training Board. She is a member of the Teaching Nurses Network in Ireland and is author of *Practical Infection Prevention and Control* (Boru Press, 2019).

**Laura Pratt (DML Training)**

Laura is a qualified Manual Handling/Patient Moving and Handling Instructor and has an MSc in Dementia Studies from Stirling University in Scotland. In 2011 Laura set up DML Training as a healthcare training business. In addition to manual handling/patient moving and handling training, DML Training also provides training in dementia care, responsive behaviour and healthcare skills in both residential and community care. DML provides training for many of the major homecare providers, a large number of residential nursing homes and educational training boards.

Laura has written chapter five (People Moving and Handling) and chapter six (People Moving and Handling Techniques).

# Contents

**1 THE DEVELOPMENT OF NURSING AS A PROFESSION**   **1**
   Irish Healthcare Service timeline   2
   History of nursing   4
   Development of nursing   8
   Industrial unrest and the Commission on Nursing   11
   Present-day nursing in Ireland   15
   Career pathways in nursing   17
   The regulation of nursing   18

**2 STRUCTURE OF THE IRISH HEALTHCARE SERVICE**   **22**
   The Department of Health   22
   Current health policy: Sláintecare   23
   Nurses in the Department of Health   24
   The Health Service Executive   24
   The structure of healthcare delivery in Ireland   26
   Nurses in the Health Service Executive   30
   Health Information and Quality Authority (HIQA)   31

**3 DELIVERING CARE**   **33**
   Nursing care   33
   Nursing values   34
   Organising care: Nursing models and frameworks   37
   The Roper, Logan and Tierney model of care   39
   The nursing process   48
   Applying the science   54

## 4 THE COMPLEX ROLE OF THE NURSE — 56

Introduction — 56
Empathy — 57
Relationships — 60
Reflection — 62
Record-keeping and reporting — 68

## 5 PEOPLE MOVING AND HANDLING — 72

Introduction — 72
Manual handling — 73
Anatomy — 75
Biomechanics — 78
Legal rights and responsibilities — 79
Safe lifting guidelines — 80
People moving and handling: the principles — 82
Communication — 91

## 6 PEOPLE MOVING AND HANDLING TECHNIQUES — 93

1. Sit to stand — 93
2. Rolling a client (roll and push) — 95
3. Slide sheets — 97
4. Hoisting — 99
5. Raising a client — 100
6. Repositioning a client — 102

## 7 INFECTION PREVENTION AND CONTROL — 104

Infections — 104
What is infection prevention and control? — 105
Micro-organisms — 106
Cross-infection — 108
Standard precautions — 111

## 8 INFECTIOUS ILLNESSES — 125

Blood-borne viruses — 125
Healthcare-associated infections — 127
Transmission-based precautions — 132

## 9 FLUID BALANCE — 137
- Normal fluid balance — 137
- Dehydration — 138
- Fluid overload — 139
- Measuring fluid balance — 140
- Fluid balance practice — 143

## 10 PHYSIOLOGICAL OBSERVATIONS — 147
- Observations/Vital signs — 147
- Measuring and recording body temperature — 148
- Measuring and recording a pulse — 155
- Measuring and recording respiration — 158
- Pulse oximetry — 160
- Measuring and recording blood pressure — 161
- Early warning system (EWS) — 166

## 11 ETHICS AND CODES OF PROFESSIONAL CONDUCT — 168
- What is ethics? — 168
- Codes of nursing ethics — 171
- Values in nursing and midwifery — 174

## 12 MEDICATION MANAGEMENT — 176
- Introduction — 176
- Legislation — 177
- Guidance on medication administration — 178
- Safety in the administration of medications — 184
- Recording and documentation — 188
- Medication errors — 188

## 13 SCOPE OF PRACTICE — 190
- Introduction — 190
- Determining the scope of nursing and midwifery practice — 193
- Scope of Practice Decision-Making Flowchart — 194

## 14 COMMONLY USED TERMS IN HEALTHCARE — 196
- Medical terms — 196
- Abbreviations — 197

## GLOSSARY — 206

## REFERENCES — 209

## APPENDICES — 215

    Appendix 1 Roper, Logan and Tierney Assessment Sheet — 215
    Appendix 2 Fluid Balance Chart — 218
    Appendix 3 INEWS Chart — 219
    Appendix 4 Medication Chart — 220

## INDEX — 221

# The Development of Nursing as a Profession

In this chapter you will learn about:

* The history and development of nursing as a profession
* The influence of European directives on nursing
* Legislation relevant to nursing
* The regulatory body for nurses and midwives
* Changes that have occurred in nursing education and training
* Societal and economic changes that have influenced nursing practice
* Present-day nurse education and training programmes in Ireland
* Present-day career pathways for nurses and midwives in Ireland

# IRISH HEALTHCARE SERVICE TIMELINE

**NURSING STUDIES THEORY AND PRACTICE**

**MIDDLE AGES:** First documented nurse was St Catherine of Siena, who practised in Santa Maria della Scala in Rome, Italy. **Care of the sick was provided mainly by religious communities and by untrained nurses of low social standing.**

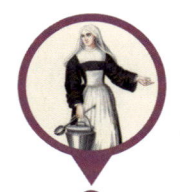

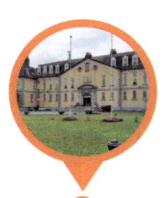

**17TH CENTURY:** Time of Enlightenment – recognition of logic and science and its significance for humanity formed the basis for health science

**1718:** First voluntary hospital, Jervis St Hospital (the Charitable Infirmary), founded, followed by others in Cork, Limerick, Waterford and Belfast

**1720:** Dr Steevens' Hospital, Dublin, is opened.

**1845–52:** The Great Famine – 1,000,000 died, 1,000,000 emigrated.

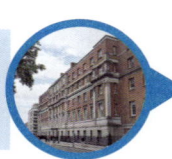

**1853–56:** Crimean War and the development of military nursing. Florence Nightingale alongside nurses recruited from Britain and Ireland Ireland and the Irish Sisters of Mercy cared for the sick and injured soldiers of this War.

**1862:** Poor Law (Amendment) Act – workhouse, infirmaries and fever hospitals converted into general hospitals

**1880:** Hospitals offer on-the-job training for nurses, which follows the Nightingale model.

**1894:** The National Maternity Hospital, Holles St Dublin, is opened.

**1897:** Irish Local Government Board – recommended appointment of trained nurses

**1900:** Nurse training formalised with apprenticeship-style training

**1918:** Midwives (Ireland) Act – formation of Central Midwives Board

**1999:** Nurses Strike

**1999:** EU Directive – length of theoretical instruction for nurse trainees to be at least one third of the training period

**2002:** First entrants to 4-year BSc (Hons) Nursing programme

**2004:** The Health Act – establishing the Health Service Executive (HSE)

**2006:** First BSc (Hons) Nursing graduates

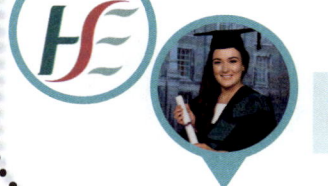

**2011:** Nurses Act

**2012:** The Nursing Board of Ireland becomes the Nursing and Midwifery Board of Ireland, recognising midwifery as a separate and distinct profession to that of nursing.

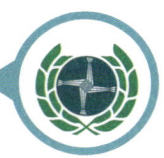

**2013:** EU Directive – revised nursing competencies

**2018:** Crisis in recruitment and retention of nurses and midwives

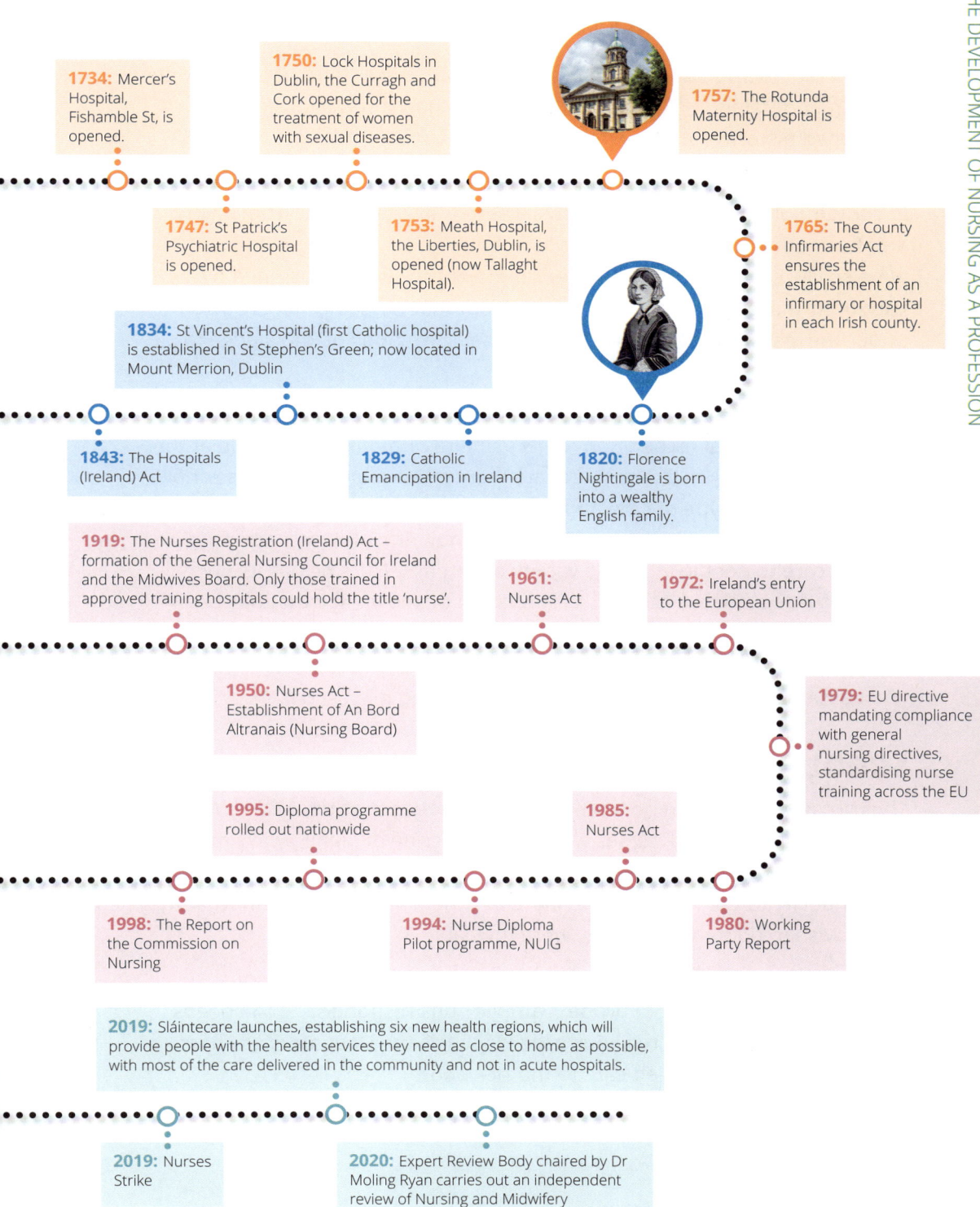

# THE DEVELOPMENT OF NURSING AS A PROFESSION

**1734:** Mercer's Hospital, Fishamble St, is opened.

**1750:** Lock Hospitals in Dublin, the Curragh and Cork opened for the treatment of women with sexual diseases.

**1757:** The Rotunda Maternity Hospital is opened.

**1747:** St Patrick's Psychiatric Hospital is opened.

**1753:** Meath Hospital, the Liberties, Dublin, is opened (now Tallaght Hospital).

**1765:** The County Infirmaries Act ensures the establishment of an infirmary or hospital in each Irish county.

**1834:** St Vincent's Hospital (first Catholic hospital) is established in St Stephen's Green; now located in Mount Merrion, Dublin

**1843:** The Hospitals (Ireland) Act

**1829:** Catholic Emancipation in Ireland

**1820:** Florence Nightingale is born into a wealthy English family.

**1919:** The Nurses Registration (Ireland) Act – formation of the General Nursing Council for Ireland and the Midwives Board. Only those trained in approved training hospitals could hold the title 'nurse'.

**1961:** Nurses Act

**1972:** Ireland's entry to the European Union

**1950:** Nurses Act – Establishment of An Bord Altranais (Nursing Board)

**1979:** EU directive mandating compliance with general nursing directives, standardising nurse training across the EU

**1995:** Diploma programme rolled out nationwide

**1985:** Nurses Act

**1998:** The Report on the Commission on Nursing

**1994:** Nurse Diploma Pilot programme, NUIG

**1980:** Working Party Report

**2019:** Sláintecare launches, establishing six new health regions, which will provide people with the health services they need as close to home as possible, with most of the care delivered in the community and not in acute hospitals.

**2019:** Nurses Strike

**2020:** Expert Review Body chaired by Dr Moling Ryan carries out an independent review of Nursing and Midwifery

3

# History of nursing

To understand and appreciate nursing and its current status, it is helpful to have an understanding of where it began and how it has evolved and developed historically.

Nursing and midwifery are distinct and separate professions. This is the case in contemporary healthcare systems, where they are distinct from each other and from other disciplines, but it was not always so. For much of history they were so closely associated with medicine that they were subsumed by it. Lack of formal education and training meant that nurses generally acted under the instruction of medics, lacking their own body of knowledge to guide their practice.

Nursing has grown in knowledge and skill and is now a profession that has gained international recognition for its value to humankind. The role of the nurse is no longer just to assist and augment medical practice; nurses now provide a specific type of care and support underpinned by their own unique knowledge. Nurses are valued members of multidisciplinary teams that provide care to people in a wide variety of settings. Nursing has its own specific value system, based on a foundation of knowledge that has been built through scientific research and analysis. The nurses of today work independently, think critically and pride themselves in providing compassionate care to individuals when they need it.

## MIDDLE AGES

The roots of nursing can be traced back at least as far as the Middle Ages. One of the first documented nurses was Saint Catherine of Siena, who practised in the hospital of Santa Maria della Scala in Rome. Saint Catherine was renowned for her ability to put herself in the place of others and do for them what they would wish to do for themselves, were they able.

During this period, care for the sick was provided mainly by religious communities. Throughout Europe, Catholic nuns responded to the needs of the sick and hurt, and religious orders such as the Daughters of Charity of St Vincent de Paul provided care to the sick poor.

## 1600–1700

During the European Enlightenment period of the late seventeenth and early eighteenth centuries, often referred to as 'the age of reason', philosophers and scientists recognised the importance of logic and science and used their learning to progress humanity. This renewed thinking encouraged the exploration of logical and scientific theories and formed the basis of health science as we now understand it (Nolan 2005).

During the post-Enlightenment period of the eighteenth century, a number of hospitals were established in Britain and in Ireland. In Britain, infirmaries were established in Manchester, Leeds, Bristol and elsewhere. Hospitals founded in Dublin in this period included Dr Steevens' Hospital, Mercer's Hospital and the Meath Hospital. The majority of these were charity hospitals.

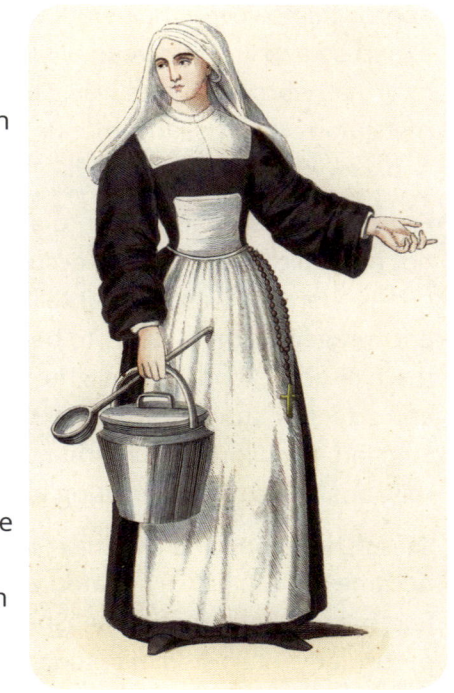

## 1800s

In the nineteenth century in mainland Europe and in Ireland, care for the sick continued to be provided predominantly by female religious orders. Mary Aikenhead, who founded the Religious Sisters of Charity in the early 1800s, established St Vincent's Hospital in Dublin in 1834. During the same era Catherine McAuley founded the Sisters of Mercy, who were extensively involved in caring for the poor and sick in Dublin (Nolan 2013).

### FLORENCE NIGHTINGALE

Military nursing also developed at this time and this is largely attributable to the work of Florence Nightingale, an English nursing pioneer who travelled to Scutari in modern-day Turkey to care for sick and injured soldiers fighting in the Crimean War (Bostridge 2008). She recruited nurses from Britain and Ireland to assist her there. The Irish Sisters of Mercy played a key role in caring for soldiers alongside Florence Nightingale. Although the sisters had little formal training, they had years of experience in caring for and visiting the sick and poor in Ireland. They were noted for their efficiency and for their caring approach; however, their work went largely unrecognised at the time. The expertise and knowledge they built up was passed from nurse to nurse in an informal, word-of-mouth way. Florence Nightingale, in contrast, kept meticulous records, documenting the care that was provided to her patients and everything she observed.

Florence was born in 1820 into a wealthy English family. In that era women did not pursue careers, instead occupying themselves with domestic and social duties. Florence was highly intelligent, and she and her sister were encouraged by their father to be critical in their thinking. He also educated them at home, and was delighted with Florence's aptitude for mathematical and scientific subjects. The Nightingale family were members of the Church of England, and Florence's mother, Fanny, took responsibility for her daughters' religious instruction, nurturing in them a strong Christian faith.

During her teens and twenties Florence became increasingly frustrated with her life and felt that she had no purpose. She was not particularly interested in getting married, but she was very interested in healthcare and nursing. Working on an intermittent basis to care for the poor in her local parish, she developed a burning desire to nurse and believed that she had been called to service by God. Although her parents had encouraged her education, they actively discouraged her from following her dreams to nurse. At the time nursing care was informal in England and there was no structured training for nurses. Nursing care was generally provided by women of the lower social classes, who were often considered to be slovenly and of poor moral character, not by educated, middle-class women. Florence's parents, therefore, considered nursing to be beneath Florence and discouraged her from pursuing her dream.

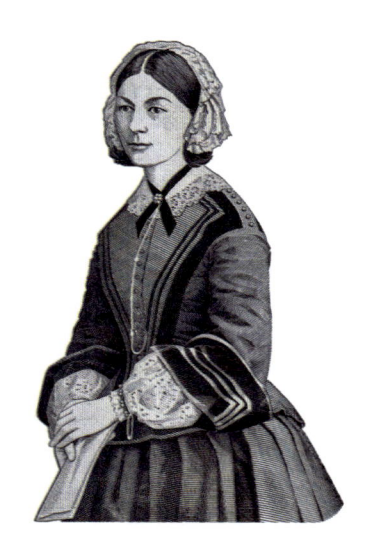

However, Florence's desire to answer her calling to care for the sick continued into her thirties. It was only when her parents witnessed her becoming depressed and became worried that that she might harm herself that they eventually permitted her to go to Germany to spend some time in one of the few nursing training schools that existed. This school, the Institute of Kaiserswerth, was in Düsseldorf and was run by Pastor Fliedner and his wife, Caroline. Here they trained deaconesses, a type of Protestant sisterhood that was becoming popular at the time among middle-class women who wished to become nurses.

Florence's thinking was ahead of its time. In her seminal work, *Notes on Nursing: What it is and What it is Not*, she speaks of nursing as aiding the reparative process of nature through the proper use of fresh air, light, warmth, cleanliness, quiet and the proper selection and administration of diet (Nightingale 1992). She described nursing as the care that puts the patient in the best possible condition for nature to act. An essential feature of nursing is what she termed 'sound and ready observation'. This is a process that focuses on all parts of the body, taking into account the fact that sometimes patients cannot speak for themselves. Nightingale believed that through controlling the environment, providing a wide range of personal services, careful observation and taking charge, the nurse aids the reparative process of nature.

Florence Nightingale was hugely influential in all aspects of nursing, in part due to her social standing in England. On her return from the Crimean War she initiated the idea that all nurses should undergo formalised training.

Nightingale sought to move away from the system of pauper nurses – untrained women who worked mostly in workhouses and cared for the sick poor. They were often elderly women who had been patients in the workhouses themselves, and although they were unpaid, they usually received some sort of recompense, such as food or liquor, for their work. Florence believed that if a more organised system of training for nurses were provided, the importance of nursing care would be more widely recognised.

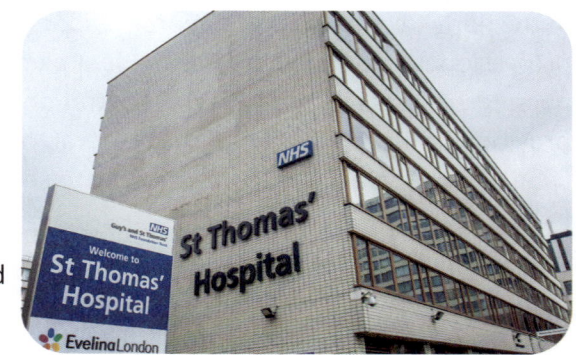

Florence is considered to be the founder of modern nursing. In 1860 she established the world's first nursing school to be continuously connected to a fully serving hospital, that of St Thomas' in London. This nursing training programme became a model for many similar training schools throughout Europe.

# Development of nursing

Until 1880, as in Britain, nursing care in Ireland was provided by untrained nurses of low social standing. Official reports of the time highlighted the deficiencies in the training of Irish nurses, and from 1880 onwards most of the larger voluntary hospitals in Dublin were required to provide 'on the job training' for nurses. In these hospitals, trainees paid a fee to enter the training programme. These reforms altered the class base of nursing and rendered it an acceptable area of professional work for middle-class women. From the late nineteenth century, nurse training in Ireland evolved and developed along the same lines as that in Britain, mainly following the Nightingale model.

## 1900s

In 1900 nurse training in Ireland was formalised and an apprenticeship-style of training developed for nurses. When recruited by a hospital, student nurses engaged in in-house education and training. They were paid service employees and constituted the majority of the workforce in Irish hospitals, so much so that hospitals depended on them to function efficiently.

In the early twentieth century nurse leaders were calling for reform and professional regulation. In 1919 the first piece of legislation in relation to nursing was passed: the Nurses Registration Act 1919. This legislation provided for the formation of the General Nursing Council for Ireland. The council, once established, had the duty to set up and keep a register of nurses in Ireland.

The development of this statute-based system of self-regulation that requires nurses and midwives to be eligible for inclusion on a register provided the basis for the characterisation of nursing and midwifery as professions (O'Shea 2013).

Nursing had become a fully regulated profession and only those nurses trained in an approved training hospital could hold the title 'nurse'. This was a significant step forward for nursing and the wider public. The Nurses Acts of 1950, 1961 and 1985 retained this register and formalised the authority under which nurses could practise.

**Bord Altranais agus Cnáimhseachais na hÉireann**
Nursing and Midwifery Board of Ireland

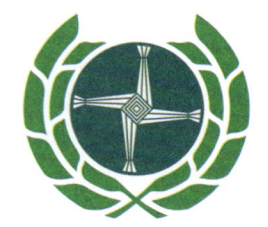

The Nurses Act 1950 established An Bord Altranais, the Nursing Board, a single entity that replaced both the General Nursing Council and the Midwives Board (Robins 2000). This board was responsible for the education, registration and professional regulation of nurses. Under the most recently published Nurses Act (2011), it is now called the Nursing and Midwifery Board of Ireland (NMBI) and still has those responsibilities.

Throughout the twentieth century, an apprenticeship style of training in hospitals prevailed in Ireland. Nurse training was a form of paid employment for young women rather than a form of higher education. Nursing remained out of mainstream education, which hindered its development, and there were vast numbers of trained, skilled, inexpensive care workers in the healthcare system.

There was constant debate among nurse educators about the ratio of practical to academic training. Nursing needed to adapt to the many influences that affected it – cultural, economic and technological. The need to increase the time spent 'off the job' and in the classroom was identified, and it was becoming more widely accepted that better educated and more skilled nurses would provide better patient care.

However, there was an economic concern. If more time during training was to be allocated to theoretical learning, the workforce in the hospitals would be depleted, and employing more qualified nurses would be more expensive. As student nurses constituted the largest proportion of people delivering care in hospitals, increasing their time in the classroom and subsequently decreasing the number of low-paid workers in hospital would cost more, and this in itself gave rise to opposition.

During the twentieth century there were other social and economic changes that were influential in nursing. Ireland's entry to the European Economic Community (now the European Union) in 1972 brought about much change in Irish society. In particular, European legislation on more equal pay and better working conditions for women was significantly influential for nursing, as it was, and remains, a predominantly female profession.

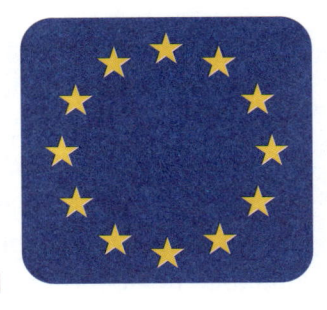

A move towards standardising nurse training across the EEC was implemented in full following the 1977 EEC Directive (implemented in 1979) that mandated compliance with general nursing directives (EEC 1977). This meant that education and training programmes across all EEC states would contain the same syllabus and student nurses would reach the same level of competency. Subsequently there would be mutual recognition of a nursing qualification across all member states. Nurses could now train and qualify in any EU state and practise in all.

In Ireland, the 1977 European Directive prompted the need to extensively examine the system of education and training for nurses. A working party was set up to do this and it took into consideration changes in society and in healthcare structures and delivery. The working party issued a wide-ranging report in 1980 and the recommendations made in this report influenced the development of nursing in subsequent years (DoH 1980).

The Nurses Act 1985 facilitated the implementation of the recommendations of the 1980 working party report. Changes were made to the structure of the Nursing Board (An Bord Altranais); membership of the board was increased; a central applications board was established so that prospective student nurses applied to the board rather than to individual hospitals; the register of nurses was divided in line with other European states; and the board had greater power to stipulate the educational requirements for entry into nurse training programmes. A Fitness to Practice committee was appointed to investigate cases of professional misconduct.

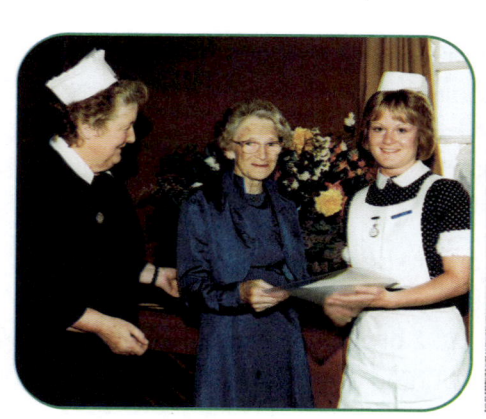

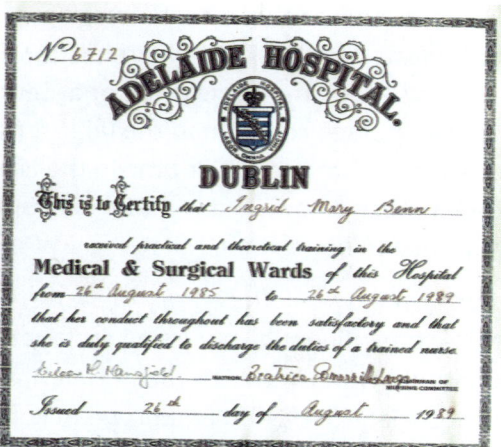

*The author receiving her qualification in 1989*

The importance of education was a central theme in the recommendations of the working party report. The working party had examined the need for university degree courses in nursing and recognised their importance. Although the report identified the need to balance practise in the clinical area with learning in an educational setting, the financial implications of reducing student nurses' time in practice and increasing their time in the classroom continued to hinder the development of a modular training system. The service needs of the hospital continued to be prioritised over the educational needs of student nurses and the apprenticeship system of training remained. Nurse training in Ireland continued as a three-year hospital-based apprenticeship model. It consisted of classroom instruction and practical training under the direction of nurse tutors in the training hospital. Assessment was continuous with preliminary and final examinations in medical and surgical nursing conducted by the Nursing Board.

A subsequent European Directive of 1989 specified that theoretical instruction should be 'balanced and co-ordinated with clinical instruction' and that 'the length of the theoretical instruction (be at least) one third and the clinical instruction (at least) one half of the minimum training period'. As an EEC member state, Ireland was compelled to comply with the directive and the 'block' study time was increased to forty weeks per student. It was generally accepted by nurse educationalists that the influence of the EU was positive for the development of nursing in Ireland.

One such positive development was the introduction, following a review by the Nursing Board, of the pilot diploma programme, which was trialled at University College Galway in 1994, in association with the National University of Ireland. This marked the beginning of a radical change in the system of nurse education and training in Ireland. The diploma programme included an increased theoretical component; the student received a non-means-tested grant rather than being paid for work performed; and students had supernumerary status in clinical areas rather than being counted in the workforce numbers. The pilot programme was considered a major improvement and over the next four years the traditional apprenticeship model was replaced with the new diploma programme nationwide. This was the beginning of links between schools of nursing and third-level institutions.

## Industrial unrest and the Commission on Nursing

Throughout the 1990s there was considerable unrest among nurses about the conditions under which they were employed. They felt that they had been flexible and had adapted to changes in technology and medical science as well as the increasing demands that changes in society had brought about. As a result of the changes in nurse training, the demands on nurses in hospitals were greater. Student nurses were supernumerary, which meant that qualified nurses had to take on some of the activities that the students had previously done. The new training system also meant that the teaching portion of the qualified nurse's role was more formalised and more demanding. Nurses felt that, as a profession, they did not get adequate recognition for the valuable work they did and the service they provided to the general public, and they felt that their level of pay and limited options for career progression reflected this.

In 1997, nurses and midwives voted for strike action, which, had it gone ahead, would have been the first time in the history of the state that nurses had gone on strike. The Labour Court, involved in the negotiations between the nursing unions and the government, recommended that government set up a Commission on Nursing to examine and report on the role of nurses in the health services. This averted strike action. The commission was chaired by High Court judge Mella Carroll and it undertook the most comprehensive review of nursing and midwifery ever seen in Ireland. It looked at:

* the evolving role of nurses, reflecting their professional development and their role in the overall management of services
* promotional opportunities and related difficulties
* structural and work change as appropriate for the effective and efficient discharge of that role
* the requirements placed on nurses, both in training and in the delivery of services
* training and educational requirements
* the role and function of the Nursing Board.

The commission's report, published in 1998, provided a comprehensive framework for the development of the nursing and midwifery professions into the future. It made over two hundred recommendations, including the following:

* The establishment of a nursing education forum to advance the transfer of pre-registration nursing education into third-level institutions at degree level
* The establishment of a national council responsible for developing relevant postgraduate education programmes
* The development of a graded structure of nurse management: clinical nurse managers 1, 2, 3

* The development of clinical career pathways: clinical nurse specialists and advanced nurse practitioners

* The introduction of the health care assistant as a member of the healthcare team to 'assist and support the nursing and midwifery function'

* The introduction of legislation to amend the Nurses Act 1985, in order to place the safety of the public at the centre of professional regulation for nursing and midwifery.

The government accepted the 197 non-pay-related recommendations, but not the three pay-related recommendations. These would have to be considered in the context of any future public service pay agreement. Nurses and their unions were disappointed with the government's refusal to implement all the recommendations of the commission. They had held back on industrial action in 1997 in the hope that their demands would be met. Now, the unions held a ballot, and an overwhelming mandate was given for industrial action. Negotiations continued between the nursing unions and government, which refused to look at pay issues outside existing public service pay policy.

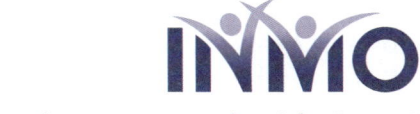

Stalemate continued and the union and its members prepared for the first all-out national strike by nurses and midwives in Irish history. A nine-day strike with only emergency services left operational took place in October 1999. After nine days of industrial action and six days of negotiations the Irish Nurses' Organisation's executive council agreed that its members should accept the Labour Court's recommendations. Information meetings were held across the country and the recommendations were accepted by the nurses and midwives in a two-thirds majority vote.

This industrial action, along with the success of the diploma programme, helped to secure the implementation of the four-year degree programme, and in 2002 the first entrants began their undergraduate programmes in universities and institutes of technology across Ireland. General nursing had changed from a three-year training programme to a four-year programme. This meant that in 2005 there were no graduate nurses eligible for registration with the regulatory body, An Bord Altranais.

Nursing practice continued to adapt to social changes. The Catholic Church became less influential on peoples' health choices as Irish society became more secular. With higher rates of immigration, Ireland became a more diverse society. Life expectancy increased at an unprecedented rate between 2001 and 2010 and as a result the number of people in Ireland aged over 65 years grew significantly.

Changes in lifestyle and behaviours brought about increased incidence of chronic diseases. Levels of type 2 diabetes, heart disease and obesity increased. Social problems such as homelessness and increased levels of drug use and addictions all impacted on the role of the nurse in Irish society.

The care that nurses provide is dynamic and evolves to meet individual needs as well as the range of needs that societal change brings about. Throughout the first decade of the twenty-first century, nurses continued to strive to improve their working conditions in line with the demands that an ever-changing society and economy placed on them. In 2006 they successfully negotiated a reduction in their weekly working hours from 39 to 37.5 hours, in line with the working hours of other healthcare professionals. However, in September 2008, only three months after the implementation of the reduced working week, economic disaster hit Ireland. The economy crashed and the government made the decision to act as guarantor to the banks. Ireland was forced to enter into a financial arrangement with the International Monetary Fund and a period of economic recession began that saw cuts across all areas of public service pay and working conditions. From 2008 to 2013, nurses experienced pay cuts, a return to a 39-hour week and a recruitment embargo that resulted in a depletion of nursing numbers across all sections of the health service.

Although pay restoration began in 2014, the impact of the economic crisis on the nursing profession was profound. The majority of newly qualified nurses were emigrating, and a recruitment and retention problem ensued as a result.

Over the next number of years working conditions for nurses continued to be challenging. The health service became more and more stretched, and issues with overcrowding in acute hospitals impacted significantly on nurses as they tried to maintain safe staffing levels in the acute hospital sector in particular. More and more nurses were emigrating and fewer were returning home from abroad.

The issue of recruitment and retention reached crisis point in 2018. A strike was held for improved pay conditions, to attract nurses into the Irish system as well as to improve the quality of patient care provided. Nurses sought pay parity with other health service grades, for example physiotherapists and occupational therapists, as they were educated to the same level and felt they had equal or greater responsibility in their role. So, for the second time in Irish history, nurses took to the picket line and the Irish Nurses and Midwives Organisation (INMO) scheduled a series of one-day strikes.

There were three days of strike action over a two-week period starting in January 2019, followed by a rally of tens of thousands of people in Dublin on Saturday 9 February. The government was reluctant to give any special consideration to the pay and conditions of nurses for fear of encouraging industrial unrest among other public sector workers and stated that it would not do anything that would undermine the current public service agreement. However, there was huge support from the general public for nurses and midwives.

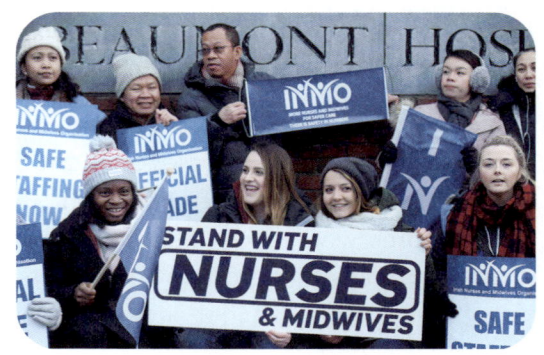

Following the mass demonstration the government held talks with the union, negotiated by the Labour Court. Strike action was suspended following recommendations by the court, which included making changes to salary scales and allowances, the promise of increased training and education opportunities and the establishment of an expert group to examine remaining pay and reform issues. Following a nationwide ballot of nurses and midwives the changes to pay were accepted and the independent review group was established. Chaired by Dr Moling Ryan and comprising members with national and international expertise, at the time of going to print the review group has yet to issue its report.

# Present-day nursing in Ireland

Nursing is currently offered as a four-year undergraduate honours degree across the universities and institutes of technology in Ireland. Prospective students apply to nursing courses through the Central Applications Office, as per the application process for other third-level courses.

There are forty-four pre-registration honours degree programmes in Ireland. These programmes lead to a specific registration: general nursing, intellectual disability nursing, psychiatric nursing, integrated children's and general nursing and midwifery.

All forty-four programmes are Honours Bachelor degree programmes at Level 8 on the National Framework of Qualifications (NFQ). The academic award is Bachelor of Science (BSc) Honours Nursing.

The four-year programme includes sixty-three weeks of theoretical instruction, forty-five weeks of clinical instruction and a final internship of thirty-six weeks' clinical placement. On completion of the programme candidates are eligible for registration.

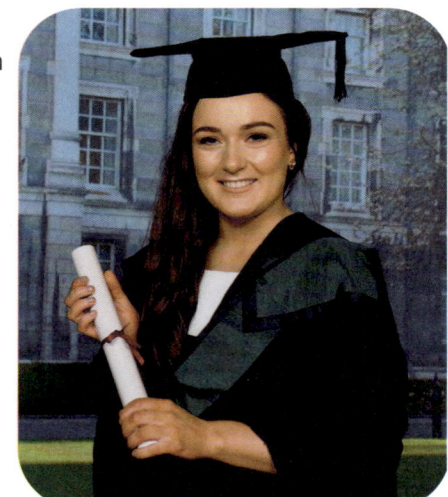

Qualified nurses can undertake a range of postgraduate courses that will enable them to progress their career. There are seven post-registration programmes leading to an additional registration with the Nursing and Midwifery Board of Ireland (NMBI).

The NMBI provides information to prospective student nurses when considering their career choices.

### Exercise

Take NMBI's student nurse/midwife self-assessment questionnaire to explore whether your interests, abilities and expectations match the role of a student nurse or midwife. The questionnaire can be found in the education section of the NMBI website (https://www.nmbi.ie/Careers-in-Nursing-Midwifery/Becoming-a-Nurse-Midwife).

Every year the NMBI publishes a careers booklet that provides information to Leaving Certificate students, post-Leaving Certificate students and mature applicants interested in becoming a nurse or a midwife (NMBI 2021).

Current undergraduate programmes leading to registration with the NMBI:

* General Nursing – 4-year programme
* Intellectual Disability Nursing – 4-year programme
* Midwifery – 4-year programme
* Psychiatric nursing – 4-year programme
* Integrated Children's and General Nursing – 4.5-year programme

Postgraduate courses can be undertaken to gain registration in other areas of nursing. The register contains twelve divisions in Ireland. Nurses and midwives may be registered in more than one division of the register.

*Divisions of the Register of Nurses and Midwives*

| Division | Designation Title | Abbreviation |
| --- | --- | --- |
| General Nurses Division | Registered General Nurse | RGN |
| Midwives Division | Registered Midwife | RM |
| Children's Nurses Division | Registered Children's Nurse | RCN |
| Psychiatric Nurses Division | Registered Psychiatric Nurse | RPN |
| Intellectual Disability Nurses Division | Registered Nurse Intellectual Disability | RNID |
| Public Health Division | Registered Public Health Nurse | RPHN |
| Nurse Tutors Division | Registered Nurse Tutor | RNT |
| Midwife Tutors Division | Registered Midwife Tutor | RMT |
| Nurse Prescribers Division | Registered Nurse Prescriber | RNP |
| Midwife Prescribers Division | Registered Midwife Prescriber | RMP |
| Advanced Nurse Practitioners Division | Registered Advanced Nurse Practitioner | RANP |
| Advanced Midwife Practitioners Division | Registered Advanced Midwife Practitioner | RAMP |

# Career pathways in nursing

Registering and practising as a nurse is just the beginning. Nursing is a career with a diverse range of opportunities. Nurses generally choose one of the following career trajectories; however, it is possible to move between them:

* **Clinical** – for nurses who are interested in a specific area of healthcare and who want to work directly with patients and clients. They usually gain experience in that area after qualification and then consider taking a

postgraduate course. This would allow them to move along the clinical career pathway and they may become a clinical nurse specialist (CNS) or an advanced nurse practitioner (ANP).

* **Management** – for nurses who enjoy organising and co-ordinating care. This role involves managing and supervising staff. Managers usually progress through clinical nurse manager 1, 2 and 3. Additionally, there are assistant director of nursing (ADON) roles and director of nursing (DON) roles.

* **Education and research** – these roles can be in universities, institutes of technology or centres of nursing and midwifery education attached to hospitals. Research pathways may be within a clinical role or nurses can work as researchers in a variety of research facilities.

Developments in nursing and midwifery since the Commission on Nursing have included an increase in nurse- and midwife-led services, the involvement of nursing and midwives in prescribing, and major changes in the demands being placed on nurse and midwife managers (O'Shea 2008).

# The regulation of nursing

Nursing and midwifery in Ireland are regulated by the Nursing and Midwifery Board of Ireland (NMBI). The role of the board is to promote high standards of professional education, training, practice and professional conduct among nurses and midwives (NMBI 2016).

The board is mandated by legislation to set standards and requirements for the initial professional education of registered nurses and midwives, which provide guidance for higher education institutions on the education of registered nurses across the divisions of the register. The standards and requirements were most recently reviewed in 2016, in order to meet revised nursing competencies as set out in the EU Directive of 2013 (EU 2013). Regular review of the content of nurse education programmes is necessary as the role of the nurse is dynamic and is influenced by changes in demographics and in healthcare delivery. In Ireland we have an ageing population, and in recent years there has been an increased emphasis on primary and community care. These changes influence the role of the nurse in society.

The NMBI maintains the register of nurses and midwives and is responsible for compliance with EU directives relating to nursing and midwifery. It provides guidance to nurses by setting practice standards.

The board is also responsible for the regulation of nurses. As part of its aim of protecting the public, it investigates complaints made by patients, their families, healthcare professionals, employers or other nurses and midwives. A full investigation into a complaint is carried out by the Fitness to Practice committee, which then issues a report. The report will contain the findings of the investigation and the decisions made by the committee. This may involve the imposition of sanctions on the nurse, e.g. a censure, an admonishment, the attachments of conditions, temporary suspension of practice, or cancellation of the nurse's registration (NMBI 2017).

The recommendation by the Commission on Nursing to introduce legislation to amend the Nurses Act 1985 in order to place the safety of the public at the centre of professional regulation for nursing and midwifery took twelve years to implement. At the end of 2011, the Nurses Act 1985 was replaced by the Nurses and Midwives Act 2011. The Act brought to an end a period of self-regulation for the profession that had stretched from 1919 to the end of 2011. It represented a radical overhaul in the way in which nursing and midwifery are regulated, with a new emphasis on public safety and accountability and the introduction of a lay majority board.

Under the current legislation the regulation of nurses and midwives continues to be the responsibility of the NMBI, whose primary responsibility is the protection of the public in their dealings with nurses and midwives. Under previous legislation the board consisted of twenty-nine members, seventeen of whom were nurses elected by nurses. The Minister for Health appointed the other twelve members, one of whom was to be a nurse. This meant that at any one time at least eighteen of the twenty-nine members were nurses. The 2011 Act brought about changes to the structure of the board. The new board is smaller, consisting of twenty-three members, eleven of whom are either registered nurses or registered midwives. The remaining twelve members are not nurses or midwives; therefore nurses are now outnumbered on the board by people who are not from the profession. The Fitness to Practice committee also has a majority of members who are not nurses or midwives (Van Dokkum 2011).

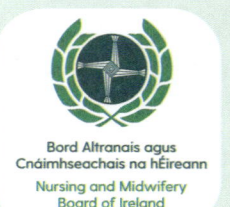

The NMBI comprises twenty-three non-executive members and a number of committees and sub-committees that report to the board. The NMBI is managed on a day-to-day basis by the chief executive officer (CEO). Five departments support the work of the office of the CEO and are led by members of the senior management team. These departments are:

* Registration
* Fitness to Practice
* Education
* Corporate Services
* Careers.

The legislation requires the board to make rules in relation to the operation of its main functions. The Nursing Rules of 2010 and 2013 provide the framework for the implementation of the legislation. Some new rules were added in 2018.

## Key legislation/EU directives

Nurses' Registration Act 1919

Nurses Act 1950

Nurses Act 1961

Nurses Act 1985

Nurses and Midwives Act 2011

1979 EU Directive

1989 EU Directive

2013 EU Directive

## REVISION QUESTIONS

1. Outline the key differences between the old 'apprenticeship' style training for nurses and today's training programme.
2. List the key pieces of legislation that have influenced the development of nursing in Ireland.
3. In what year was the Nursing Board (An Bord Altranais) established?

4. Describe the influence of EU directives on the development of nursing.
5. Outline the events that led to the establishment of the Commission on Nursing.
6. What were the main recommendations of the Commission on Nursing Report 1998?
7. Outline some social and economic changes that have influenced the development of nursing practice.
8. List the current divisions of the Register of Nurses and Midwives in Ireland.
9. Consider the three career pathways listed on pages 17–18. Which might you like to follow? Explain your choice.
10. Outline the three main functions of the Nursing and Midwifery Board of Ireland.
11. Outline the changes to the structure of NMBI that followed the most recent Nurse Act, and describe the impact of those changes.

# Structure of the Irish Healthcare Service

In this chapter you will learn about:

* The function of the Department of Health
* Current healthcare policy
* The role of nurses at the Department of Health
* The function of the Health Service Executive (HSE)
* Members of primary, secondary and tertiary healthcare teams
* The role of nurses at the HSE
* The Health Information and Quality Authority (HIQA)

## The Department of Health

The Department of Health is responsible for policy development in Ireland. Its mission is to improve the health and wellbeing of people in Ireland by: keeping people healthy; providing the healthcare people need; delivering high-quality services; and getting best value from health service resources. The department's role is to provide strategic leadership for the health service and to ensure that government policies are implemented effectively. The department supports the ministers of state in their implementation of government policy and in discharging their duties.

> ### Exercise
>
> Carry out your own research to identify the current minister for health in Ireland and the other ministers of state at the Department of Health. Outline which area(s) of health each minister is responsible for.

## Current health policy: Sláintecare

Sláintecare, introduced in 2017, is a ten-year blueprint for the reform of the health service. It is the first time in Ireland that there has been political consensus on a health reform plan across all political parties. The plan provides a vision for a new health service that will deliver a universal health system in Ireland. Provision of healthcare is funded by general taxation and everyone in Ireland is provided for under the current system. However, in the past we have seen the development of a two-tier system of healthcare delivery: the publicly funded system; and a private system funded through private investment and private health insurance. Historically, where waiting lists to access care have grown within the public system, people who can afford private health insurance have done so to avoid having to wait for essential care and to ensure they get what they consider to be better-quality care. A two-tier system such as the one that currently exists in Ireland is less equitable than a universal system of healthcare provision and it is one in which access to care is based on the ability to pay rather than on need.

Sláintecare aspires to provide:

* entitlement for all Irish residents to all health and social care
* no charges to access GP, primary or hospital care
* care provided at the lowest level of complexity, outside hospital, in an integrated way
* eHealth as a tool for integrating care
* a strong focus on public health and health promotion

* shorter waiting times to access care
* private care phased out of public hospitals
* better mental health services
* an expanded workforce
* a new HSE board
* ring-fenced funding for health.

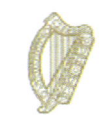

An Roinn Sláinte
Department of Health

## Nurses in the Department of Health

In Chapter 1 we discussed the development of nursing as a profession. Nurses in Ireland now play a key role at all levels of healthcare delivery. At the Department of Health, the Office of the Chief Nursing Officer provides professional policy direction and evidence-based advice. The office works to ensure that nurses and midwives have input at government level. The perspective of nurses and midwives is vital in ensuring that their skills are used to the full extent and that the professions are as flexible as possible to cope with the ever-changing health needs of people living in Ireland.

The chief nursing officer is responsible for the provision of strategic leadership and expert nursing and midwifery advice to the Department of Health, government, the broader health system and regulatory and professional bodies. Their responsibilities include professional regulation, workforce planning and allied healthcare professionals.

### Exercise

Carry out your own research to identify the current chief nursing officer at the Department of Health.

## The Health Service Executive

The Health Service Executive (HSE) is responsible for policy implementation and service delivery. The current healthcare system in Ireland is governed by the Health Act 2004. The HSE was established under this act on 1 January 2005.

The HSE replaced the previous system, which comprised ten regional health boards. Until 2019, the HSE was divided into four administrative regions; however, as part of the implementation of Sláintecare there will be six new health regions for Ireland.

The HSE's vision is to have 'a healthier Ireland with a high-quality health service valued by all'. Its core values are care, compassion, trust and learning.

The HSE's mission is to ensure that people in Ireland:

* are supported by health and social care services to achieve their full potential

* can access safe, compassionate, quality care when they need it

* can be confident that the HSE will deliver the best outcomes and value through optimising its resources. (HSE 2015a)

Map of six new health regions

The HSE takes responsibility for the delivery of all publicly funded health and social services nationally including acute hospitals, social care, mental health, primary care, health and wellbeing, and the national ambulance service. The HSE also provides community care. This is the provision of care to people outside acute hospitals, in their own community, either in their own home or in a nearby healthcare facility.

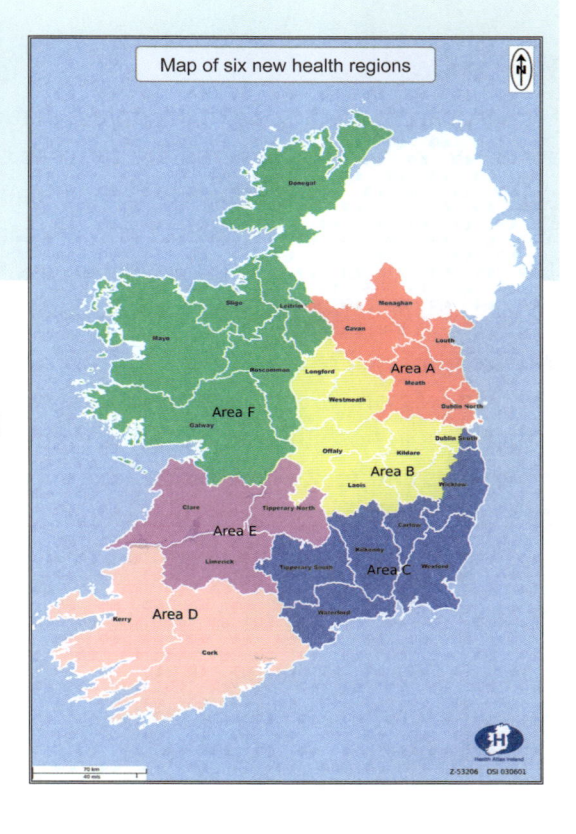

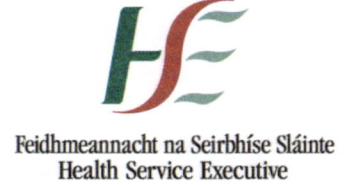

Feidhmeannacht na Seirbhíse Sláinte
Health Service Executive

# The structure of healthcare delivery in Ireland

Generally, healthcare is provided at three different levels in Ireland.

## PRIMARY CARE

Primary care is the first point of contact that people have with the health and social services. Since 2001 primary care has been the central focus of the delivery of health and social services in Ireland (DOHC 2001). It is provided in settings such as GPs' surgeries or primary care centres in local communities. The aim of primary care is to provide accessible, integrated, high-quality services to meet the needs of local populations.

Where primary care services are available, hospital-based interventions might not be necessary. It costs less to provide care for individuals in the community rather than in hospital, and it is more empowering for clients to identify their own needs and seek professional advice from an appropriate source. Primary care settings also provide an opportunity to carry out health promotion activities such as disease prevention, health education and screening activities.

### PRIMARY CARE TEAM MEMBERS

* **General practitioners (GP)** – doctors who specialise in primary care medicine. They engage in health education and promotion activities as well as screening, disease prevention, diagnostics and treatments. When a person's needs cannot be met at primary care level the GP will refer them to the relevant secondary or tertiary care service.

* **Practice nurses** – nurses who have undergone specialist training in primary care. They provide vaccinations, health screening services and nurse-led clinics. They play a key role in supporting people to manage chronic conditions, out of hospital.

* **Dietitians** – experts in food and nutrition. They provide educational and practical advice to people and act as consultants to other healthcare

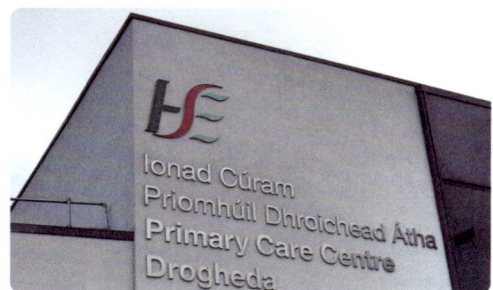

professionals. They work with target groups to provide nutritional programmes and instructional presentations.

* **Occupational therapists –** promote health and wellbeing through occupation. They work to enable people to do things that will enhance their ability to participate in activities or by modifying the environment to better support participation. They analyse physical, environmental, psychosocial, spiritual and cultural factors to identify barriers to occupation.

* **Physiotherapists –** provide services to individuals to develop, maintain and restore maximum movement and functional ability throughout the lifespan, for example where movement and function are threatened by ageing, injury, disease or environmental factors.

* **Speech and language therapists –** work with people with communication disorders to help them achieve their maximum potential. They diagnose and treat communication impairments and swallowing disorders in children and adults.

* **Chiropodists –** treat minor disorders of the feet and nails.

## SECONDARY CARE

The term 'secondary care' refers to a service provided by medical specialists who generally do not have first contact with patients, for example general consultant surgeons and physicians in acute hospitals. Referral to secondary care services is usually by a GP or through an accident and emergency department.

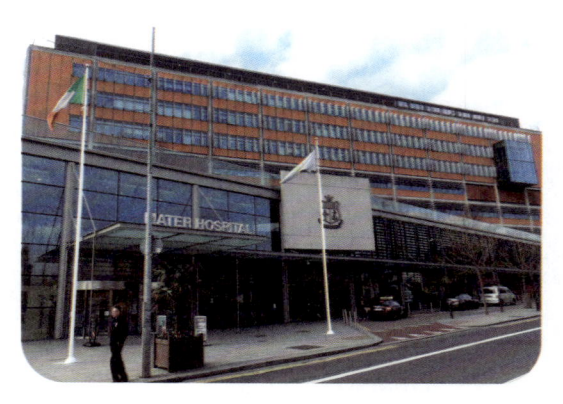

The role of secondary care is to accept referrals from primary care, to carry out relevant investigations, make a diagnosis and treat the presenting condition. Members of the secondary care team will also provide advice and information to the patient.

## SECONDARY CARE TEAM MEMBERS

* **Consultant surgeons –** engage with people who have been referred from primary care. They carry out investigations and tests to diagnose the cause of the presenting condition, and treat the person, often using surgical procedures.

* **Consultant physicians –** engage with people who have been referred from primary care. They carry out investigations and tests to diagnose the cause of the presenting condition and provide medical treatments, e.g. prescribe medications, lifestyle changes or other interventions.

* **Nurses –** provide support and nursing interventions to people in acute hospitals.

* **Health care assistants –** provide care to people under the supervision and direction of nurses.

* **Dietitians –** act as consultants to other healthcare professionals. They review medical charts, advise on nutritional therapies and treatments and offer advice to people and their families.

* **Radiologists and radiographers –** carry out X-rays and scans to assist in the diagnosis of illness and injury. They interpret the results of the investigations and provide the information to consulting surgeons and physicians.

* **Physiotherapists –** provide support to restore and maintain functional ability for people undergoing surgical or medical treatments.

* **Social workers –** provide social support to people in preparation for discharge from hospital. They intervene in crisis situations, provide protective services to vulnerable people and help people to deal with practical and financial issues.

* **Pharmacists –** ensure the safe and effective use of drugs and drug treatments prescribed by healthcare professionals. They have the responsibility of controlling supply and administration of pharmaceutical drugs in hospitals.

## TERTIARY CARE

Tertiary care is care that is provided in a healthcare facility by highly trained specialists, often using advanced technology. This is usually specialised consultative care that is provided following referral from primary or secondary medical care personnel. It is provided by specialists working in a facility that caters for special investigation and treatment, e.g. specialised cancer care, dermatology, plastic surgery, neurology, fertility care.

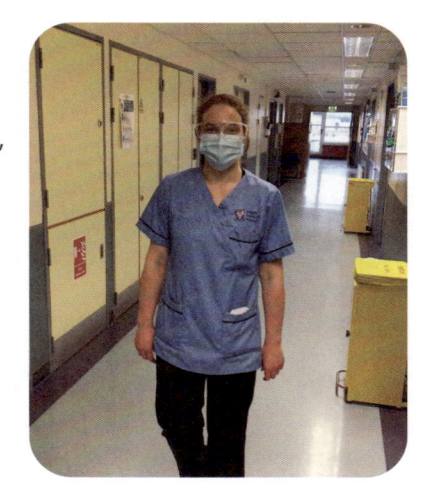

An example of tertiary care is the National Cancer Control Programme (NCCP), which has been in place since 2007 and is currently led by Professor Risteárd Ó Laoide. The programme was initially set up to map out the future of cancer treatment in Ireland. Its implementation involved the transfer of all major cancer treatment to eight designated Specialist Cancer Centres.

## SPECIALIST CANCER CENTRES

The Specialist Cancer Centres were originally located and networked within the original four HSE administration areas; this was to ensure as even a geographical spread as possible:

* Beaumont Hospital
* Mater Hospital
* St James's Hospital
* St Vincent's University Hospital
* Cork University Hospital
* Waterford Regional Hospital
* University College Hospital Galway
* University Hospital Limerick.

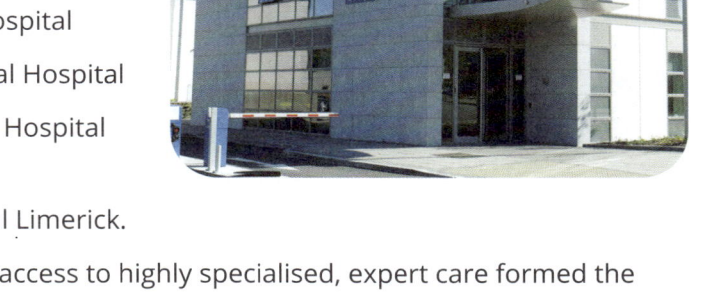

The provision of equal access to highly specialised, expert care formed the basis of the plan for this tertiary service. Currently there are seven hospital groups in Ireland and each of the hospital groups have at least one designated cancer centre. Each centre must be supported by general medical and surgical infrastructure, e.g. pathology laboratory, radiology services, rehabilitation care and palliative care, and each centre would carry out research, education programmes and specialist training.

The provision of care within these eight centres is universal and is funded through the HSE. Faster access cannot be achieved through the private system.

## TERTIARY CARE TEAM

Specialist consultants usually lead the tertiary care team. The other members of the tertiary care team share this area of expertise and include specialist nurses, dietitians, physiotherapists, occupational therapists, etc. Members of the team may be skilled in performing specialised tests and treatments that may involve using advanced technology.

## COMMUNITY CARE

Community care is the provision of care in the individual's own home. Care may be provided by staff directly employed by the HSE, e.g. public health nurses or community care assistants, or by private providers under contract to the HSE, e.g. Home Instead, Comfort Keepers.

Staff involved in community care include:

* health care assistants
* speech and language therapists
* community pharmacists
* psychologists
* chiropodists.

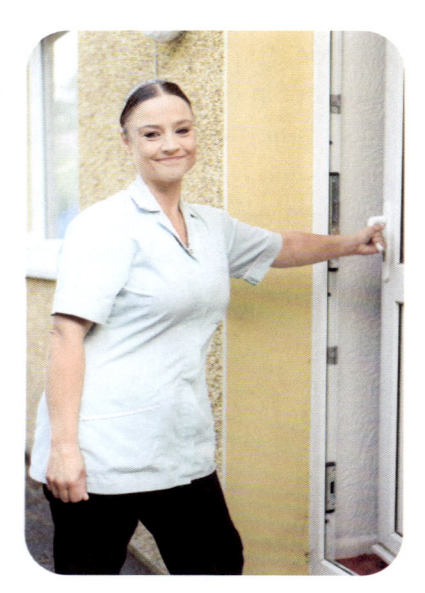

# Nurses in the Heath Service Executive

The HSE's Office of the Nursing and Midwifery Services Director (ONMSD) works to lead and support nurses and midwives in the delivery of safe, high-quality, person-centred care.

The ONMSD provides staff to lead on specific aspects of the National Clinical and Integrated Care Programmes. It promotes quality improvement and delivers guidance and expertise at corporate, regional and local level. It is a focal point for nursing and midwifery within the public health system and it provides expertise that is central to the analysis, application, implementation and evaluation of legislation and health policy relating to nursing and midwifery practice.

The ONMSD collects and analyses data that informs and supports national decision-making as it relates to nursing and midwifery and manages and co-ordinates the design, development and delivery of continual professional development for nurses and midwives.

# Health Information and Quality Authority (HIQA)

The founding principle of HIQA is to contribute to the programme for reform of the health services. It was established on an interim basis in May 2005 and on a statutory basis in May 2007. This was seen as a significant step on the road to a major improvement in the quality of health services in Ireland.

HIQA is an independent authority that reports to the minister for health and is responsible for driving quality and safety in Ireland's health and social care services.

HIQA's role is to:

* develop and set standards in health and social services
* monitor healthcare quality though a system of inspection.

According to HIQA:

> Everyone using health and social care services should be confident that their experience will be a safe one. To help deliver quality care for all, our work will focus on setting standards on safety and quality, monitoring to ensure these standards are being met and conducting investigations where there is a serious risk to the health and welfare of health or social care service users. (HIQA, 2012)

## HIQA INSPECTIONS

HIQA carries out inspections of healthcare and social services to monitor and protect vulnerable clients by ensuring that service providers are complying with legislation and national standards. HIQA can require that changes are made in line with recommendations from previous inspections to ensure the best quality of care. HIQA will also carry out an inspection if there has been a complaint about a service provider. It can carry out announced or unannounced inspections.

### Exercise

Discuss the differences between primary, secondary and tertiary care. In groups, discuss the different role that nurses play at each of these levels of care:

* Practice nurse in a primary care centre
* Nurse working on a general surgical ward in an acute hospital
* Nurse working in a medical ward in an acute hospital
* Nurse working in a tertiary burns unit
* Nurse working in an intensive care unit in a tertiary centre for cardiac surgery
* A public health nurse.

# Delivering Care

**3**

In this chapter you will learn about:

* The delivery of nursing care
* Evidence-based practice
* Person-centred care
* Holistic care
* Nursing models and frameworks for delivering care
* The Roper, Logan and Tierney model of care
* The nursing process

## Nursing care

The essence of nursing and midwifery is to provide care and support to those that need it. Nursing and midwifery are science-based professions. Practice is developed based on evidence that is generated through research. In all practice professions there has been a move away from acting on personal intuition and experience to acting on research; but what does this mean? The following example demonstrates how this translates into a nurse's practice.

### Non-evidence-based practice

When this author was a student nurse in an inner-city Dublin hospital in the mid-1980s, the prevention of pressure ulcers was a practice issue of concern to nurses. It still is today. A pressure ulcer, also called a pressure sore, can develop in people with restricted movement. An area of skin can break down when force or pressure is applied during periods of immobility, e.g. the skin on heels or elbows when lying in bed.

In each ward of the hospital the sister-in-charge would have her own theory and practice in relation to preventing the development of pressure sores. In one ward, the nurses vigorously rubbed the skin in the affected areas at two-hourly intervals to stimulate circulation. In another ward they painted egg white on the skin and dried it with oxygen, thinking that it would form a protective seal on the skin. In another, Sudocrem was rubbed into the skin of the affected area at regular intervals. These different practices were based on the individual sisters' personal opinions, experiences and often hunches. This is a far cry from the evidence-based practice that nurses engage in today.

Nowadays, nursing care and nursing interventions are based on scientific research studies that have been carried out and replicated. The results of the replicated studies are then compared and contrasted to evaluate the effectiveness of the nursing intervention.

### Gathering evidence to inform practice

If a new type of pressure-relieving mattress was introduced to prevent the occurrence of pressure ulcers in patients with reduced mobility due to stroke, research would be carried out to see how many patients developed pressure sores while using the mattress over a specific period of time. The results of that study would be compared with a similar group of patients who did not use the mattress. This research would be replicated in other stroke units and the results analysed. The analysis of this data would provide the evidence that would measure the effectiveness of the mattress in preventing pressure ulcers in people with reduced mobility due to stroke. This is a scientific method of developing nursing practice. It is what is meant by 'evidence-based practice'.

## Nursing values

In the analysis of patients' needs and the organisation of care, nursing practice has developed in a similarly methodical and scientific way. Nursing is often described as being a 'science and an art'. The practice of nursing is underpinned by scientific knowledge developed through enquiry and research. The application of that knowledge in practice is the art of nursing, and this is a complex process. The complexity arises from the fact that nursing is all about caring for people. Therefore, nursing practice must also be guided by certain principles that reflect the value that the nursing profession places on people.

## PERSON-CENTRED CARE

When we value people, we aim to provide care that focuses on the person and that recognises the importance of the person's individual needs. This is referred to as person-centred care. The person requiring care is at the centre of the planning and provision of care. The following values underpin the provision of person-centred care:

* **Individuality –** Each person is recognised as an individual with his/her own unique needs and care requirements. No two people will ever have exactly the same needs.

* **Respect –** The rights of the person are acknowledged. A procedure is never undertaken, or an action carried out, that would go against the person's wishes. The person is always listened to and given an opportunity to express their preferences.

* **Partnership –** Care provided is planned in partnership with the person. The type of care provided is agreed between the nurse and the patient with shared goals in mind. The person is always provided with information that is understandable to them so that they can make an informed decision about their care.

* **Privacy and dignity –** Every individual has the right to privacy and dignity. This includes privacy of information, which is strongly linked with the principle of confidentiality. It is also about maintaining an appropriate level of intimacy and protecting what the person values as private to them. It is important that nurses take steps to treat a person with dignity in all aspects of care.

* **Confidentiality –** Patients and clients have the right to have their personal and private affairs kept confidential. To do otherwise is an invasion of privacy. Personal information is valuable and enables the nurse to care properly for the person. This type of information is regarded as privileged and must only be passed on to a supervisor or colleagues if it is thought to affect the person's wellbeing or the wellbeing of others.

* **Independence –** Promoting maximum independence is a value that is fundamental in nursing and midwifery. An accurate assessment of needs will ensure that nurses do not provide the wrong level of care and, in doing so, cause the person to become more dependent.

* **Positive self-image** – Self-esteem reflects the value that an individual places on himself or herself, and it depends to a great extent on the way we are treated by others. Nurses have an important role to play in promoting self-esteem by helping people to feel good about themselves. This can be done by valuing and respecting their individuality and encouraging them to be independent and involved in decisions about their welfare.

* **Empathy** – Empathy is the ability to put yourself in the place of another person and to try to experience what they are experiencing. In other words, it is the act of 'putting yourself in someone else's shoes'.

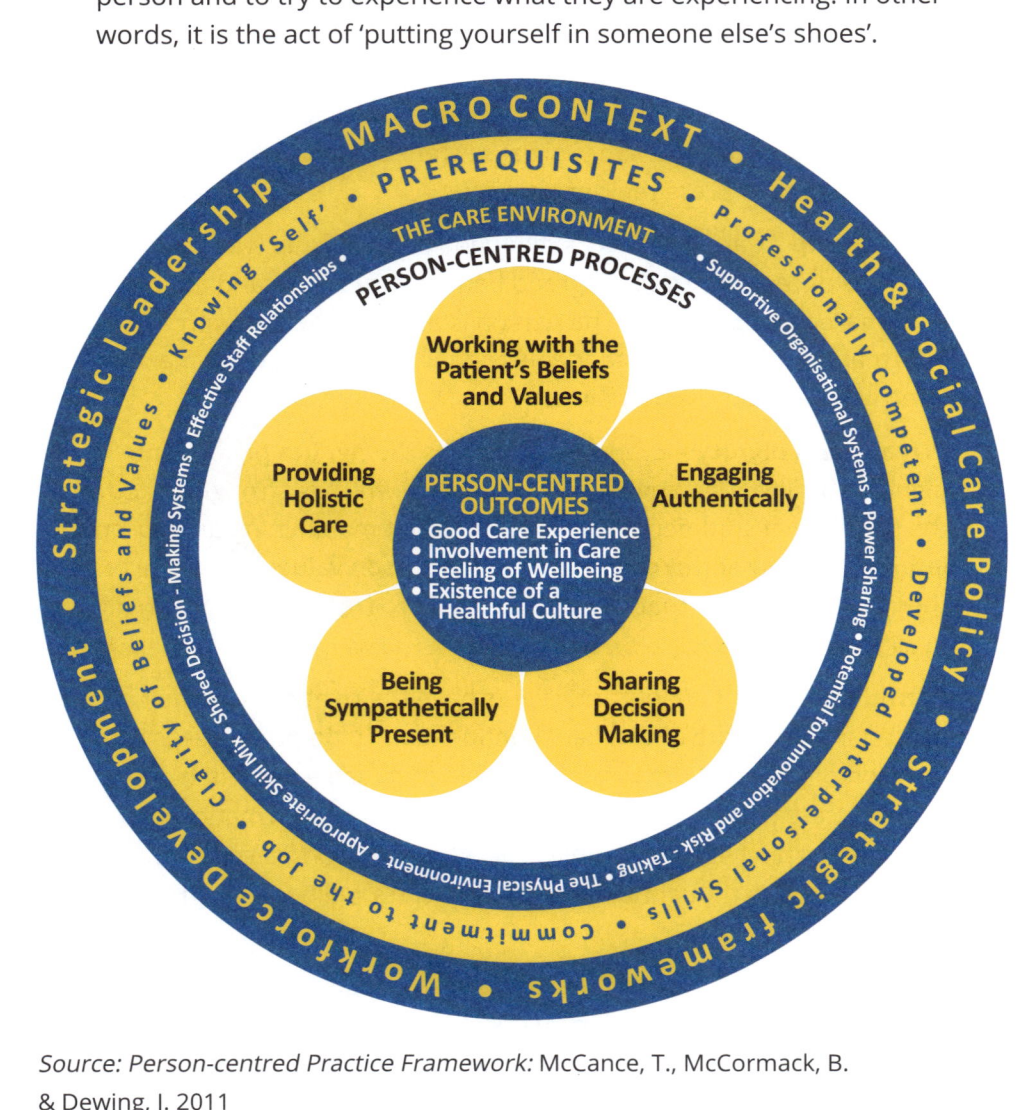

*Source: Person-centred Practice Framework:* McCance, T., McCormack, B. & Dewing, J. 2011

## HOLISTIC CARE

When nurses consider the care a person needs, they look at that person in their entirety, as a whole. If they are caring for someone who is suffering from a chronic condition such as diabetes, they don't just provide care that will keep the person's blood sugar levels within normal limits; they look at the person in the situation that they are in, including how they feel, the other people in their lives, the person's values and beliefs and the physical and financial resources available to them. This is holistic care.

# Organising care: Nursing models and frameworks

Organising and providing care to people, as you can see, is a complex process. Scientific knowledge and evidence must be considered while taking into account the principles of person-centredness. Nurses strive to meet all the needs of the person. In doing so, the theory of nursing has developed. It is the theory of nursing that provides a framework or a structure within which to provide care.

A number of nursing theorists have developed different 'nursing models' that have served as effective frameworks for developing systems for providing care.

The **Neuman model of nursing** is a conceptual framework, or a visual representation, for thinking about patients and nurses and their interactions (Neuman 2011). This model views the person as a layered, multi-dimensional whole that is in constant dynamic interaction with the environment. The layers are considered a way of protecting the core being and maintaining balance within the person and in their life. Betty Neuman theorises that two major components responsible for maintaining that balance is the stress experienced by the person and the way they react to it. She sees prevention as the main way of maintaining balance and designed a nursing model that facilitated this.

Another nursing theorist, **Patricia Benner**, takes the Dreyfus model of skill acquisition and applies it to nursing. According Benner's model, nurses progress from being novices to experts principally through the knowledge they gain in the practice of nursing. In other words, the knowledge they gain in the practical world is important for the development of the nurse's skills and ability to care (Benner et al. 1996).

The **Orem model of nursing**, also known as the 'self-care' model of nursing, was developed in 1985. It is widely used in rehabilitation and primary care settings. The Orem model is based on the philosophy that all patients wish to care for themselves. Dorothea Orem identified groups of needs or requirements, or self-care requisites. When individuals are unable to meet their own self-care needs, a self-care deficit occurs. It is the job of the nurse to determine these deficits and to find a support modality based on analysis of the dependency level of the individual.

The **Roper, Logan and Tierney model of nursing** is based on a model of living. Nancy Roper, Winifred Logan and Alison Tierney, three Scottish nurse theorists, published *The Elements of Nursing* in 1980. This work identified the individual aspects of the model as a whole and how nursing could use it as a framework for the care of patients in a wide variety of settings. This model, widely used by nurses and carers in the UK and in Ireland, looks specifically at meeting all the client's needs. It is a model that embraces person-centredness and holism.

All models involve some method of assessing patients and offering the appropriate care. A key part of the model is identifying how progress will be evaluated, so that you know if what you are doing is effectively meeting the person's needs or if you need to do something else.

Models give rise to care plans – documents that translate the care suggested into a format through which nurses can document what they are doing, and what other professionals should be asked to do. They are changed and evaluated on a daily basis and as the client's condition and abilities change.

A nursing framework is the way a nurse organises the care delivered to the client. It is based on a nursing model. There are different kinds of framework: some are on paper (e.g. assessment sheets), some are in your head (conceptual frameworks) and some are both. Do not rely on the paper frameworks alone. It's up to you as a nurse to have a clear vision for the way you approach care. Frameworks are built as an expression of the different models.

*See Appendix 1 Roper, Logan and Tierney assessment sheet (p. 215).*

# The Roper, Logan and Tierney model of care

(For convenience, this model will be referred to as Roper.)

The Roper model is divided into two parts: the **model of living** and the **model of nursing** (Holland et al 2003).

## THE MODEL OF LIVING

There are five components in the model of living:

* Activities of daily living
* Lifespan
* Dependence/independence continuum
* Factors influencing the activities of daily living
* Individuality in living.

## ACTIVITIES OF DAILY LIVING

Living is a complex process which we undertake using a number of activities to ensure our survival. They have been identified by Roper separately; however, as nurses, we cannot look at one activity to the exclusion of the others. Our daily activities are interdependent: for example, in order to eliminate, we need to eat and drink first; in order to survive to carry out any activity, we need to breathe all the time. Remember that nurses take a holistic approach to care.

## TWELVE SPECIFIC AREAS OF DAILY LIVING

* **Maintaining a safe environment:** comfort, freedom from pain, avoiding injury (e.g. falls), preventing infection and monitoring change.
* **Communicating:** verbally/non-verbally, forming relationships, expressing emotions, needs, fears and anxieties. Using smell, touch, taste, hearing, sight and sensitivity.
* **Breathing:** meeting body oxygen requirements, maintaining a clear airway and lung expansion.
* **Eating and drinking:** meeting nutritional needs, maintaining a healthy diet suitable to the individual.
* **Eliminating:** excretion of urine and faeces, maintaining normal function and control.

- **Personal cleansing and dressing:** skin, hair, nails, mouth, teeth, eyes and ears. Selecting appropriate clothing, dressing and undressing.
- **Controlling body temperature:** physically adjusting personal clothing and body covers.
- **Mobilising:** exercising for health, maintaining muscle tone and circulation, counteracting the effects of mobility, relieving pressure to skin, changing position, using mobility aids.
- **Working and playing:** activity, pleasurable pastimes, achievement, independence and partnership in care/rehabilitation.
- **Expressing sexuality:** expressing sexuality, fulfilling human needs.
- **Sleeping and resting:** adequate sleep and rest periods.
- **Dying:** acceptance of inevitability, peaceful without pain or distress, needs met, needs of loved ones met.

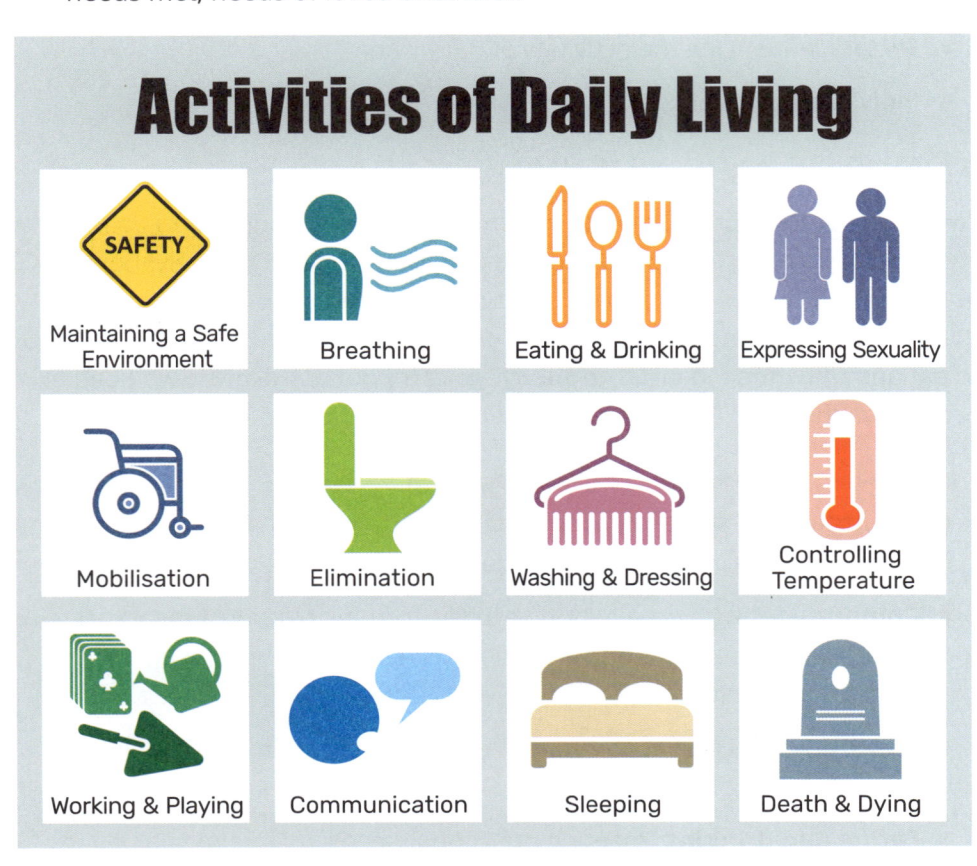

## Activities of Daily Living

| | | | |
|---|---|---|---|
| Maintaining a Safe Environment | Breathing | Eating & Drinking | Expressing Sexuality |
| Mobilisation | Elimination | Washing & Dressing | Controlling Temperature |
| Working & Playing | Communication | Sleeping | Death & Dying |

## LIFESPAN

The lifespan is a continuum indicating movement of an individual from birth to death through the different stages:

* Infancy
* Childhood
* Adolescence
* Adulthood
* Old age.

According to Roper, Logan and Tierney, 'As a person moves along the lifespan there is a continuous change, and every aspect of living is influenced by the biological, psychological, socio-cultural, environmental and politico-economic circumstances encountered through life.'

## DEPENDENCE/INDEPENDENCE CONTINUUM

This component of the model is closely related to the lifespan and the activities of daily living. It is included to acknowledge that there are stages in the lifespan when a person cannot perform certain daily activities independently. Each person is said to have a dependence/independence continuum for each activity. Their level of independence or dependence will vary over the course of their lifespan depending on events and on their age.

Take eating and drinking as an example. As a baby we depend on another person to provide food; however, we do have the ability to suck a breast or a bottle immediately after birth. As we move along the lifespan we become more independent in the activity of eating and drinking, we are able to use our hands to feed ourselves, we are able to prepare our own food, and so on.

During adolescence we would expect a person to be fully independent in their ability to eat and drink. However, imagine if the person fell off a swing and fractured both wrists – what effect would this have on their level of independence? This would be a temporary state, but it would significantly affect where they are on the continuum of independence/dependence at that time.

We will assume that they make a full recovery from their fall and return to where they were on the continuum beforehand. They progress into adulthood. In old age they have a stroke which affects their ability to eat and drink independently. They engage in stroke rehabilitation and regain some of the function they had previously and so, with assistive equipment, they can manage to eat independently.

So you can see that where we are on the continuum is dynamic and is constantly influenced not only by age but by events and circumstances throughout the lifespan. Most importantly, nurses recognise that the lifespan is a different experience for everyone, and so individuality is recognised.

*The lifespan continuum*

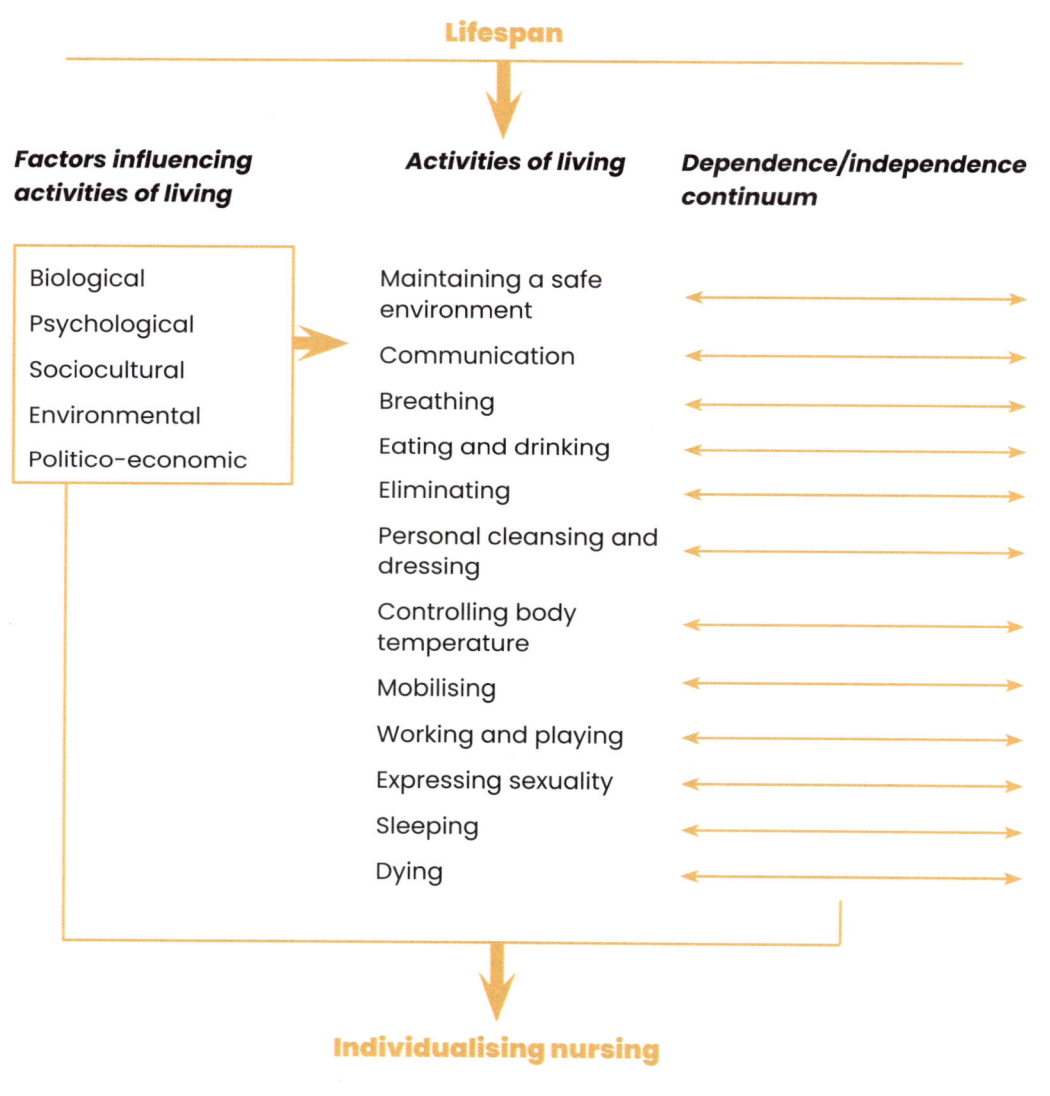

**Lifespan**

| Factors influencing activities of living | Activities of living | Dependence/independence continuum |
|---|---|---|
| Biological<br>Psychological<br>Sociocultural<br>Environmental<br>Politico-economic | Maintaining a safe environment<br>Communication<br>Breathing<br>Eating and drinking<br>Eliminating<br>Personal cleansing and dressing<br>Controlling body temperature<br>Mobilising<br>Working and playing<br>Expressing sexuality<br>Sleeping<br>Dying | ←————→<br>←————→<br>←————→<br>←————→<br>←————→<br>←————→<br>←————→<br>←————→<br>←————→<br>←————→<br>←————→<br>←————→ |

**Individualising nursing**

*Source:* Kara 2007

# FACTORS INFLUENCING THE ACTIVITIES OF DAILY LIVING

There are numerous factors that influence our daily lives and the activities we carry out. Roper, Logan and Tierney have divided them into five main categories:

* Biological
* Psychological
* Sociocultural
* Environmental
* Politico-economic.

## BIOLOGICAL

For the purpose of this model of living, the term 'biological' relates to the human body's structure and physical performance. This is strongly influenced by an individual's genetic inheritance. For example:

* A person's height is strongly influenced by their genetic make-up, but if they do not eat a healthy diet during the first part of the lifespan this may affect their growth.
* A person may be born with a specific genetic condition, e.g. if they have cystic fibrosis, this will have a significant effect on the activity of breathing.
* A person may be born with Down's syndrome – this may affect their ability to communicate or maintain a safe environment.

The lifestyle choices we make affect the body's physical condition and performance. Bad health habits can have a cumulative effect on the body, e.g. dietary habits or cigarette smoking.

## PSYCHOLOGICAL

Psychology is the study of how humans behave. How we behave is influenced by factors such as our beliefs, our thoughts and our feelings. Education influences how we develop and think about the various aspects of our life. Our experiences throughout life also strongly influence how we behave. Our emotional development is closely linked to intellectual development and lifespan. If our emotional needs are not met as a child, this will affect our behaviour throughout the lifespan. It may affect our ability to carry out several of our activities of daily living, e.g. communication, working and playing, expressing sexuality and dying.

### SOCIOCULTURAL

The society and culture in which we live will influence our intellectual and emotional development. What is considered the norm in one culture may be considered otherwise in another. Family structures and societal values strongly influence how we live our lives.

### ENVIRONMENTAL

The environment refers to the conditions experienced in the area where we live. These factors include our living conditions as well as climate, pollution, war, famine and natural disasters like flooding or earthquakes.

### POLITICO-ECONOMIC

This is very strongly linked to the country or jurisdiction in which a person lives. In Ireland we are subject to Irish law, which in turn is very strongly influenced by European laws. The laws of a country reflect the values and beliefs of the people that live there. In a democracy, individual citizens have the opportunity to express their beliefs and influence the laws that govern them through voting for public representatives and changes to laws. In non-democratic countries citizens have less power and may be subject to laws or polices that they do not believe in or agree with. The political situation in one region often leads to people fleeing and seeking refuge in another country where they believe they will be safer and have a better quality of life.

## INDIVIDUALITY IN LIVING

Roper, Logan and Tierney acknowledge that each individual will experience and carry out their activities of daily living in their own unique way. This will be influenced by the factors we have already mentioned.

## THE MODEL OF NURSING

So far, we have looked at the Roper model of nursing from the perspective of the individual. Now we will look at the model from a nursing perspective.

The following are thirteen assumptions that Roper, Logan and Tierney make about the values and beliefs of the nursing profession. These values and beliefs underpin their model of care and provide the basis for assessment and care planning.

1. Living can be described as a combination of activities of living.
2. Each person carries out their activities of living in their own individual way – this is their right.
3. The individual is valued at all stages in the lifespan.
4. Generally speaking, throughout the lifespan until adulthood, the individual tends to become increasingly independent.
5. While independence is valued and encouraged, dependence should not diminish the dignity of the individual.
6. An individual's knowledge, attitudes and behaviour related to their activities of living are influenced by a broad range of factors including biological, psychological, sociocultural, environmental and politico-economic.
7. The way in which a person carries out their activities of living fluctuates within a range of what is normal for that person.
8. When an individual is ill it may give rise to problems with their activities of living, both actual and potential. A problem, in this context, is an unmet need.
9. During the lifespan, an individual may experience significant life events which can affect the way they carry out their activities of living. These life events may lead to problems, both actual and potential.
10. The concept of potential problems includes the promotion of good health and the prevention of illness or injury.
11. In the caring context, nurses work in partnership with the individual. The individual is recognised as an autonomous, decision-making person.
12. Nurses work with other health professionals as part of a multidisciplinary team. The person being cared for is always at the centre of care delivery and the team works for the benefit of that person.
13. The specific purpose of the nurse is to assist and support the individual to prevent, alleviate, solve or cope positively with actual and potential problems related to their activities of living.

**Virginia Henderson** is another nurse who theorised about nursing and care delivery. She defined nursing as:

> The unique function of the nurse is to assist the individual, sick or well, in the performance of those activities contributing to health or its recovery (or to peaceful death) that he/she would perform unaided if he had the necessary strength, will or knowledge. And to do this in such a way as to help him/her gain independence as rapidly as possible. (Henderson 1966)

Nurses need to be knowledgeable in relation to lifespan development, the dependence/independence continuum and the factors influencing the activities of living – biological, psychological, sociocultural, environmental and politico-economic.

## LIFESPAN

From a nursing perspective, young babies and children admitted to hospital will have different needs from adults. Involvement of the family is encouraged to avoid the adverse effects of separation. The support needed by parents of a child dying from cancer will differ from those of an adult child of an older person dying from natural causes in their eighties or nineties.

The care provided to an adolescent requires an understanding of their physical and emotional development, in particular when they are faced with a serious illness such as diabetes that requires a radical alteration to their lifestyle.

The care needs of adults and older adults will depend on the reason they encounter health services. The care needs of an older person with cancer will differ from those of an older person with dementia. Knowing how to care for older people and what happens during the process of ageing is therefore an essential part of the nurse's role if they are to ensure that the care they plan to deliver will meet the individual needs of a person.

## DEPENDENCE/INDEPENDENCE CONTINUUM

This continuum is an important part of the model of nursing. It reminds us that during our lifetime we can, depending on our health and life circumstances, move from the very dependent stages of infancy and childhood to the independent adult and older person stage. Ill health or injury, however, can make us partially or totally dependent in either one or more of our activities of living. This can happen at any stage of the lifespan.

The nurse will help the individual progress towards independence in the activities of living and at other times help the person to accept dependence.

## FACTORS INFLUENCING THE ACTIVITIES OF LIVING

To be able to use the model of nursing effectively requires the nurse to have knowledge of the five factors we mentioned above and how they influence the activities of living.

* Knowledge of the structure and function of the heart (biological factors) will help the nurse to explain what happened during a heart attack, as will knowledge of the effects of smoking or obesity on the heart when promoting healthy living.
* Understanding the possible psychological effects of having a heart attack will make it easier to explain to a patient's relations how the patient is likely to respond to their illness.
* Understanding the patient's beliefs (sociocultural factors) will enable the nurse to offer the appropriate assistance with personal hygiene needs.
* Where and how the person lives (environmental factors) will be essential knowledge when considering their discharge home from hospital. Will an elderly person who has had a stroke be able to manage the stairs if they live in a two-storey house? Will a child with chronic asthma living in a damp flat be affected by their environment?
* Knowledge of social services and how the HSE works when discussing a patient's entitlements to home care (politico-economic factors) will facilitate the planning and delivery of care to an individual who needs it.

As with the model of living, the factors influencing the model of nursing interlink with the lifespan and the dependence/independence continuum to enable the nurse to adopt a holistic, person-centred approach to care.

In the following example, we can see how a nurse uses his/her knowledge of the factors influencing the activities of living to assess a person's needs.

### CASE STUDY

Jack is a 24-year-old college graduate who has hypertension. He has completed a degree in business, but he is having difficulty getting a job. All the jobs he thinks will suit him are in Dublin; however, rental properties are hard to come by and very expensive. He is back living with his parents in Roscrea, having led an independent life in Limerick for the last four years. He has a sedentary lifestyle and a BMI of 29.

| Factor | Nurse/carer's knowledge |
|---|---|
| Biological | The structure and function of the cardiovascular system. Is there a family history of coronary heart disease? What is the normal blood pressure range for Jack's age? |
| Psychological | Is Jack experiencing stress in his situation? If so, will this affect his hypertension? Is stress contributing to his BMI? He was living independently; now he has become more dependent on has parents than he was as an adolescent. |
| Sociocultural | Is this affecting his lifestyle? His eating habits? Do his family or friends take exercise? What are their eating habits? Are his peers working and living independently? |
| Environmental | Can he access healthy food from where he lives? Can he access the means to exercise? |
| Politico-economic | Are government policies contributing to his inability to get work or accommodation in Dublin? Are there any government policies/agencies that could contribute to helping him reduce his hypertension? |

# The nursing process

Each patient is unique, as is the relationship between the nurse and the patient. The Roper, Logan and Tierney model offers a framework for nurses that ensures that this individuality is taken into account when caring for a person. To make sure that all aspects of an individual's life are integrated into an effective care plan, Roper uses a problem-solving approach and the nursing process in conjunction with the model for nursing.

## THE NURSING PROCESS AND CRITICAL THINKING

The nursing process is the foundation for critical thinking. It underpins all care models and provides a tool for decision making. It is a tool for learning how to 'think like a nurse' (Alfaro-LeFevre 2014). Nurses value people as individuals and recognise their own need to be able to think critically and adapt to each different situation.

The nursing process is a critical thinking model used to promote a competent level of care provision. It gives nurses an organised, systematic way of thinking about patient care and it guides nurses' thinking.

Applying nursing process principles helps the nurse to:

* organise and prioritise patient care
* focus on what is most important – patient safety, response to care, health status, quality of care
* develop thinking habits that are needed to reason through clinical situations and make effective decisions about patient care.

There are **five phases in the Nursing Process**. Each phase is designed to achieve a specific purpose. The phases guide the nurse to think in a systematic, organised way. This helps to avoid missing anything important when providing care. The phases are:

1. Assessment
2. Diagnosis
3. Planning
4. Implementation
5. Evaluation

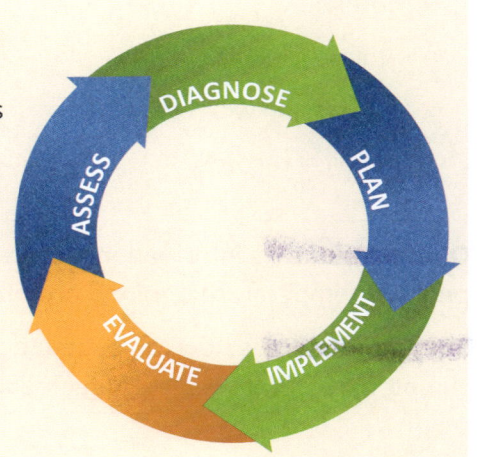

The nursing process is used with Roper, Logan and Tierney's activities of daily living framework to provide effective, good-quality care. This method of providing care can be utilised in all situations.

## 1 ASSESSMENT

Assessment should be an ongoing process rather than a once-off activity. Initial assessment is necessarily followed by regular reassessment as the patient's circumstances and condition change. Assessment involves collecting information about the person and their situation. It includes:

* collecting information from/about the person
* reviewing the collected information.

The main information comes, whenever possible, from the patient – this is referred to as a **primary source of information**. Information from family members is referred to as a secondary source. When it is not possible to collect information from the patient, e.g. if they are unconscious, secondary sources become particularly important.

Information can be collected in a number of ways and confidentiality is always an essential element of every stage of care provision.

> Methods of obtaining information include:
> * Observation
> * Interview
> * Physical examination
> * Discussion with relations
> * Medical records.

**Objective data** is information that can be observed and measured, e.g. a person's temperature or blood pressure.

**Subjective data** is how the patient defines or reports their own experience, symptoms and feelings, e.g. 'I feel really hot', 'My stomach really hurts'.

### Exercise

Imagine you have tonsillitis. Identify what objective data would be gathered about you by the nurse and what subjective data you would describe.

The purpose of collecting information relevant to each activity of living is to discover:

* previous routines
* what the person can do independently
* what the person cannot do independently
* previous coping behaviours
* what problems the person has, both actual and potential.

> **Remember!**
> In this context, a problem is an unmet need.
> An **actual problem** is an unmet need that exists now,
> e.g. not being able to drink independently.
> A **potential problem** is something that could occur in the future as a result of that need not being met, e.g. dehydration.

> **Exercise**
>
> In a group, go through the twelve activities of daily living and identify actual and potential problems that could occur in different care situations.

## 2 DIAGNOSIS

This involves analysing data collected during assessment to determine a nursing diagnosis. Be careful not to confuse a nursing diagnosis with a medical diagnosis. In making a diagnosis the nurse is trying to determine: if there are risks for safety or infection transmission; what the actual and potential problems are for the person; and the priorities among problems – sometimes the nurses' priorities and those of the patient may differ. The nurse draws conclusions about signs and symptoms that may need to be evaluated by another member of the multidisciplinary team, e.g. the physiotherapist or dietitian, and makes the referral. The nurse identifies whether the person has any learning needs; and the strengths and resources that the person has that will enable them to address their problems.

## 3 PLANNING

Care is planned according to the nature of the actual and potential problems that are identified. The plan depends on the nurse's knowledge of appropriate care to be given for that health problem, taking into account the individuality of the patient.

According to Roper, Logan and Tierney, the purpose of the plan is as follows:

* Preventing identified potential problems becoming actual problems
* Solving actual problems

- Alleviating those problems that cannot be solved
- Helping the patient to cope positively with problems that cannot be solved or alleviated
- Preventing recurrence of a treated problem
- Helping a person to be as pain-free and comfortable as possible when death is inevitable
- Developing strategies for support and resources and referring to other healthcare professionals
- Working collaboratively and co-operatively, identifying who else might need to be involved in the person's care
- Identifying what the person will need for discharge home (if an in-patient)
- Identifying if any equipment, aids or adaptations are needed, either in the clinical environment or at home and how the person will access the required equipment, etc.

To achieve the plan requires the nurse and the individual to set goals, both short term and long term, for the actual and potential problems that were identified during assessment. Remember that a partnership approach to care is taken. Good communication and interpersonal skills are required for successful planning. A therapeutic relationship where the person has trust in the nurse is a vital component of effective planning.

Some goals will be for the nurse to achieve and some will be for the patient to achieve. For example, if a patient has high blood pressure it is the nurse's goal to ensure that it is measured regularly and that the prescribed medication is administered. On the other hand, if the patient is very anxious about the blood pressure it could be his goal to discuss his anxiety with the nurse and engage in some activity that will help to reduce the anxiety.

Setting and achieving goals will depend on the patient, the health problems and the resources available.

In addition to planning care and setting goals through verbal and non-verbal interaction between the nurse and the patient it is necessary to document all stages of the nursing process. This is essential for continuity of care and it provides documentary evidence that good quality care is being provided.

Nurses and carers work as part of a multidisciplinary team and so all members of the team should have access to the patient's records.

The nursing care plan should contain the following:

- Stated goals or desired outcomes for each problem
- An expected time frame for achieving the stated goals
- The planned nursing interventions and patient participation to achieve the goal.

## 4 IMPLEMENTATION

Implementation is the next stage of the nursing process and it involves putting the plan into action. The nursing interventions or actions are carried out. The actual problems are dealt with and potential problems are prevented.

The nurse provides the right level of care and support, encouraging the person towards maximum independence. During implementation, the nurse is listening and talking, observing and measuring, teaching and promoting good health. The nurse may be providing treatments, medications or therapies. The person and the nurse will be working together and in some case with others too.

The nurse may be supporting the person to cope when it is not possible to solve actual problems. This may mean helping someone to cope with the fact that they may not get better or that death is inevitable.

## 5 EVALUATION

The purpose of evaluation is to assess how effective the care provided has been in meeting the person's needs. If there has been inaccuracy in the assessment stage it will affect the diagnosis, planning and implementation of care and this can be identified during evaluation.

Evaluation can be carried out by:

- observing
- questioning
- examining
- testing
- measuring.

Have the implementations been effective or ineffective? Has the person benefited? Are they progressing towards independence? Have the goals for actual problems been met? Were the potential problems prevented? Does the plan need to be modified? Has anything that should have happened not been done?

To a large extent the evaluation reflects the accuracy of the assessment, the appropriateness of the planning and the effectiveness of the implementation.

*The Nursing Process: A Summary*

| Stage | Activity |
|---|---|
| Assessment | Continuously collecting data about health status to monitor for evidence of health problems and risk factors that may contribute to health problems (e.g. smoking) |
| Diagnosis | Analysing data to identify actual and potential problems, risk factors and strengths |
| Planning | Determining desired outcomes (benefits expected to be seen in the patient after care) and identifying interventions to achieve outcomes |
| Implementation | Putting the plan into action and observing initial responses |
| Evaluation | Determining how well the outcomes have been met and deciding whether changes need to be made; looking for ways to improve things |

*Source:* Alfaro-LeFevre 2014

# Applying the science

Nursing is often referred to as both a science and an art. In this chapter we have looked at the science behind providing care for people. We know that the models and frameworks that nurses use as tools to ensure the provision of safe, effective care are evidence-based. They have been tried and tested by nurses all over the world and it is in the application of these tools to practice, in real life situations, that the real skill or art of nursing can be seen.

When students undertake clinical placements, they have the opportunity to use these scientific theories. Initially they observe other nurses doing so and then they start to participate in care provision themselves and apply their knowledge to care for people. This is where the joy of nursing happens.

In preparation for clinical placements it can be extremely useful to practise applying the nursing models and frameworks to case studies. Have a go at doing this with the following two case studies.

## CASE STUDY

Mary is a 79-year-old woman who has just been admitted to your ward. She has osteoarthritis of the hips and asks you to assist her to the bathroom. Apply the nursing process to the mobility activity of daily living to describe the care that you provide to Mary.

## CASE STUDY

Jordan is a 19-year-old boy who has broken his right arm playing rugby. He had a plate and pins inserted in his arm in theatre yesterday and his arm is in a cast. It is breakfast time, and he needs assistance to eat.
Apply the nursing process to the eating and drinking activity of daily living to describe the care that you provide to Jordan.

# 4

# The Complex Role of the Nurse

In this chapter you will learn about:

* The difference between sympathy and empathy
* Empathic behaviour using a person-centred approach
* Building an empathic relationship in nursing
* The role of advocacy in empathic behaviour
* Different types of advocacy
* Reflective practice in nursing
* Record-keeping and the role of the nurse in clinical practice

## Introduction

The role of the nurse is complex. Becoming a nurse requires a wide range of skills and abilities. Nurses need to be able to understand complex scientific principles and to apply those principles in a practice. They need to be able to do this in a way that embraces the value of human kindness and caring. They need to have a level of emotional intelligence that enables them to interpret the feelings and needs of the people they care for. All of this has to be done in the context of contemporary healthcare, where nurses are morally and legally responsible and accountable for both their actions and their inactions. In this chapter we are first going to look at some of the 'soft skills' that are required to fulfil the role of the nurse and then we will look at the importance of precision and accuracy in recording the care that is provided.

# Empathy

Empathy is the ability to imagine yourself in the place of another person and to try to experience what they are experiencing – 'putting yourself in someone else's shoes'. This is different from sympathy, which involves feeling sorry for another person.

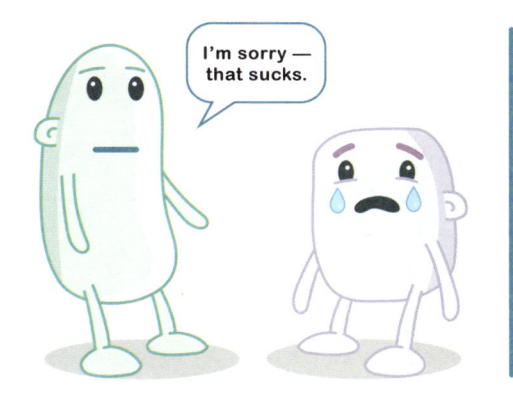

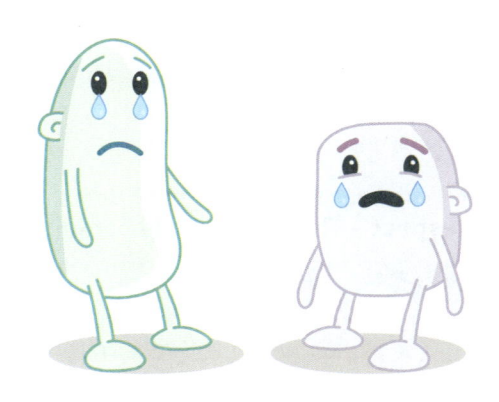

### DEFINITIONS

**Sympathy** – the verbal and non-verbal expression of sorrow or dismay.

**Compassion** – active participation in another individual's suffering.

**Empathy** – an understanding not only of the other's beliefs, values and ideas but also the significance that their situation has for them, and their associated feelings. (Chowdhry 2010)

Nurses incorporate empathy into every action they take and every interaction they have with the people they care for and their families. How a nurse makes a person feel is as important as the task that is being carried out. It is important that nurses have an appreciation of the impact that their actions and reactions have on people and how they feel.

Communication and interpersonal skills play a really important role in conveying empathy. A reassuring smile, an acknowledgment of distress or the use of therapeutic touch can make a person feel that they matter and that they are understood. Lack of empathy can make a person feel worse about their situation, unimportant and disempowered.

Being mindful of the principles of person-centred care that underpin nursing practice will help us to be empathic towards people.

Examples of actions that nurses can take to convey empathy, using a person-centred care approach, include:

**Individuality –** Each person is recognised as an individual.

| Action | Impact |
| --- | --- |
| Introduce yourself to the person and know their name before you approach them | The person feels that they are important to you and that you do not view them as 'just another patient' |
| Respect the person's preferences for food choices | Choice allows a person to express their individuality |

**Respect –** The rights of the person are acknowledged.

| Action | Impact |
| --- | --- |
| Use body language to actively listen to the person when they are telling you something | The person feels that they are being listened to and that their feelings matter |
| Never carry out an action without first gaining the person's consent. If they refuse, accept their decision. | The person is empowered and feels in control of their situation |

**Partnership –** The care that is provided is planned in partnership with the person.

| Action | Impact |
| --- | --- |
| Discuss the person's problems and possible solutions with them | The person feels that they are making their own decisions, not that they are being made for or about them |
| Discuss the goals of treatments with the person | The person feels that they have something to work towards and there is hope for improvement in the person's situation |

**Privacy and dignity –** Every individual has the right to privacy and dignity.

| Action | Impact |
| --- | --- |
| When assisting someone with their personal hygiene, make sure only the part of the body that is being washed is exposed and not their whole body | They will feel less embarrassed. Being completely exposed feels very undignified. |
| Facilitate the practice of religious or cultural beliefs | The person feels able to express themselves in their preferred way; this will give them comfort |

| Action | Impact |
| --- | --- |
| Don't enter a person's room or bedspace without first knocking or seeking permission | There is no invasion of privacy; the person feels ownership of their space |

**Confidentiality –** Patients and clients have the right to have their personal and private affairs kept confidential. To do otherwise is an invasion of privacy.

| Action | Impact |
| --- | --- |
| If you need to have a confidential talk with someone, make sure that you do it in a room where there is privacy and not in a ward where others can hear | The person will feel valued and this will increase their trust in you |
| Allow a person privacy when they are on a phone call or have visitors | The person feels able to talk to their loved ones in a safe and private space |

**Independence –** Promoting maximum independence is a value that is fundamental in nursing and midwifery.

| Action | Impact |
| --- | --- |
| Allow the person to do as much as they can for themselves. This may take longer than providing assistance, but it is important not to rush the person or do anything that will make them feel rushed | The person gains confidence and feels they are progressing |

**Positive self-image –** Self-esteem reflects the value that an individual places upon himself/herself, and it depends to a great extent on the way we are treated by others.

| Action | Impact |
| --- | --- |
| Facilitate the person to choose their clothes for the day and to wear their preferred jewellery | The person feels well presented to the world for the day and feels good about themselves |
| Ensure a client's glasses are accessible or their hearing aid is in full working order | Not being able to see or hear properly makes a person feel more vulnerable and less in control of their situation |

## Exercise

Write down what would be important to you if you were dependent on others for assistance with your activities of daily living.

Discuss with your classmates how that would make you feel.

List, in order of priority, the activities that would be most important to you to perform independently.

# Relationships

The relationship between the nurse and the person being cared for is essential to the effective delivery of care. Communication and interpersonal skills occur in the context of a therapeutic relationship between the nurse and the person. The focus of this relationship is person-centred rather than task-centred. This relationship is fundamentally different from our social relationships.

Social relationships are based upon friendships whereas therapeutic relationships are based upon professional values. This requires the nurse to set aside biases, prejudices and very often their own emotions, although these personal aspects are also important as they bring compassion to the encounter that is crucial to a professional relationship.

As we've seen, empathy is a vital part of the therapeutic relationship; without empathy it is difficult for nurses to understand the needs and wants of others. When trying to empathise with others it is necessary to observe verbal signs and body language as well as an individual's external appearance and signs – such as smiling or sighing – or facial expression to gauge how they feel. However, empathy also involves trying to share and understand something internal – another person's feelings, instincts or worries. It can be difficult to decode the external and internal signs that lead to empathic understanding. If a nurse has not experienced an event or has had a different experience of a similar situation, or has little life experience, empathising can be challenging.

**Unconditional positive regard** is another vital component of the relationship. Nurses work with a wide range of people from many different social circumstances, with varying beliefs and values around health. The nurse is completely accepting towards the person and this is demonstrated through attitude and behaviour. The person feels they can disclose their emotions and concerns without fear of judgment or rejection. Nurses value the worth of every person they engage with. Everybody deserves the same level of care.

## WHAT IS A THERAPEUTIC RELATIONSHIP?

* The nurse has the responsibility to help the person regain a state of health.
* The person and the nurse negotiate and agree the level of formality.
* The focus of the relationship is on the needs of the client.

* The participants may not know or even like each other.
* The nurse seeks to be non-judgmental.
* Personal or intimate information is shared in one direction only, from the client to the nurse.
* The feelings of the client are identified and acknowledged in discussions.
* The feelings of the nurse are focused on an empathic response.
* The nurse takes responsibility for setting the boundaries of the relationship.

## ADVOCACY

The NMBI's *Scope of Nursing and Midwifery Practice* framework (2015) states, 'nursing practice involves advocacy for the rights of the individual patient and for their family. It also involves advocacy on behalf of nursing practice in organisational and management structures within nursing.'

> **DEFINITION**
>
> **Advocates** are people who speak on behalf of those whose voices are not heard. Patient advocacy is a key part of nursing practice.
>
> The NMBI defines **advocacy** as: 'a means of empowering people by supporting them to assert their views and claim their entitlements and, where necessary, representing and negotiating on their behalf'.
>
> (www.nmbi.ie/Standards-Guidance/Glossary)

Nurses advocate for the people they care for. This involves supporting the person's needs, wishes and preferences, even if they are different from those of the nurse. The foundation for advocacy is empathy, understanding what a person is experiencing. For example, if a person is undergoing a painful procedure, the nurse understands that the experience of pain is a negative one and therefore the patient will require some form of pain relief. When a person is fully conscious and in full control of their lives, they can ask for pain relief; however, this is often not the case, and when people are unable to speak up for themselves it is the role of the nurse to advocate on their behalf. This may happen in a number of situations, for example when a person has an altered level of consciousness following a traumatic injury; when a person has reduced cognitive ability due to dementia; when a person has an intellectual disability and is unable to speak up for themselves; when a person has a speech impediment following a stroke. The nurse empathises with the patient and in doing so they gain an understanding of what the person is experiencing. Then they speak up on behalf of the person and ensure that they are provided with effective pain relief.

In order to advocate for a person, the nurse needs excellent communication and interpersonal skills. Nurses work within multidisciplinary teams and often represent the wishes of the person to the other members of the team.

The therapeutic relationship that the nurse has with the person also lays the foundation for advocacy, because in order to advocate for somebody the nurse must first know what the person's wishes are. Advocacy often involves courage; in some situations you need to be brave to speak up for people and their rights. When people's basic human rights are not being met it is the role of the nurse to speak up for them, either for an individual or for people collectively. The industrial action that nurses took in 2019, in an attempt to secure safe staffing levels in acute hospitals, is an example of this type of advocacy.

Altruism – acting for the benefit of others – is a fundamental value of nursing and midwifery and so advocacy is an essential part of expressing that value in practice.

# Reflection

Reflection involves looking back at an experience or an event and the impact that it has had on us. Informal reflection is part of our everyday lives. When we buy a new food product, for example, we reflect on what it was like to eat, how it compared to other similar products, whether it was more or less expensive than other brands, and whether we would buy it again. If we watch the first episode of a new TV series, we reflect on it afterwards. Was it enjoyable? Was it too violent? Will we watch the second episode? We reflect while we are doing things too. We may love the new food product and savour every mouthful. We may not enjoy the TV programme and stop watching halfway through. These are examples of how we reflect on our everyday actions, and these reflections determine what we do next time. We are usually seeking a good experience and trying to improve things for ourselves. We are trying to find tastier food products and more entertaining things to watch on TV.

In nursing, the fundamental aim of reflection is to improve the care that is being provided. We carry out this type of reflection in a more formalised way.

When we use formal frameworks to reflect on our practice we get better and better at it until eventually it becomes second nature to us.

Nurses reflect while they are doing things, which is referred to as **reflection in-action**; and they also reflect on things after they have happened, which is **reflection on-action** (Schon 1991).

Reflective practice is an approach that promotes autonomous learning, which aims to develop students' understanding and critical thinking skills. Reflection involves looking back at an incident, thinking about what was good and what was bad about it, trying to understand it and giving consideration to how it could have been done better or how it could be done better in the future. Reflection is a very effective method of continuously improving practice and the quality of care that is being provided.

In nursing and healthcare, structured frameworks are very useful in guiding the reflective process. Gibbs' reflective cycle is one that is commonly used by nursing students and by nurses (Gibbs 1998). Remember, we never get to a point where we know everything. Every day brings new experiences.

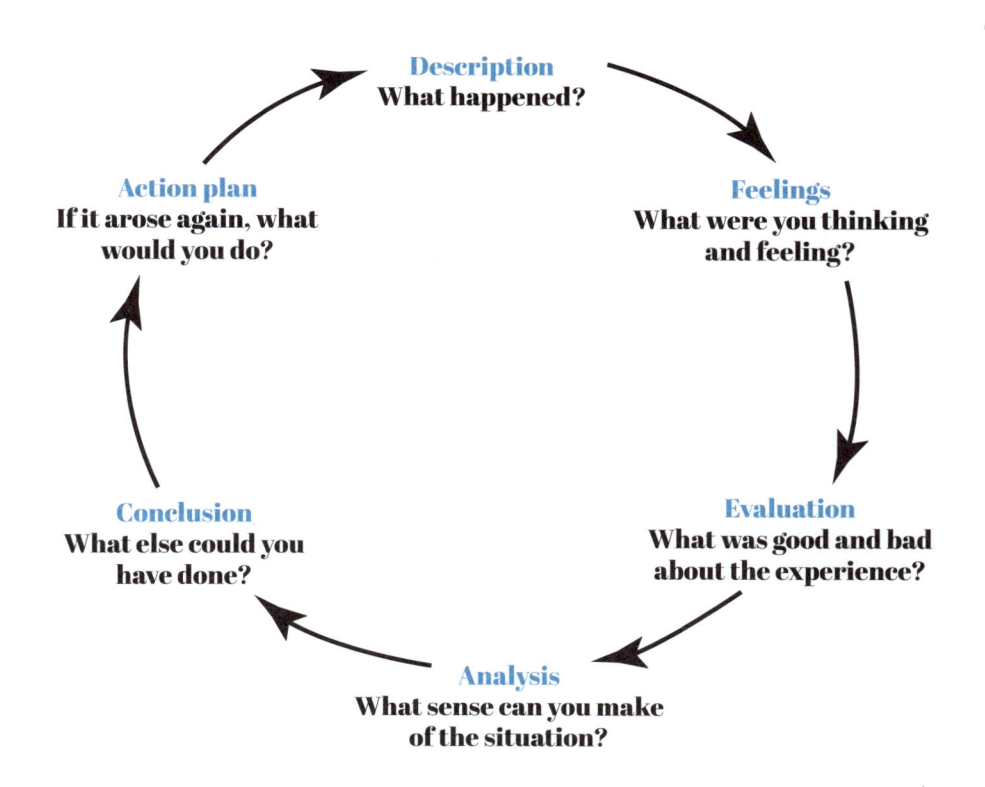

**Description**
What happened?

**Feelings**
What were you thinking and feeling?

**Evaluation**
What was good and bad about the experience?

**Analysis**
What sense can you make of the situation?

**Conclusion**
What else could you have done?

**Action plan**
If it arose again, what would you do?

| | |
|---|---|
| **Description – of the event/what happened** | A significant event happened to me today <br><br> The most important event that happened to me at work/work experience today <br><br> Thinking back over the day <br><br> Whilst reflecting on my work experience day |
| **Feelings – What was I thinking and feeling?** | I felt so surprised by my feelings of <br><br> One of the things that surprised me was <br><br> It was so shocking when <br><br> I was so upset when <br><br> I felt quite embarrassed when <br><br> I feel happy that <br><br> I was frustrated when <br><br> I was positive when |
| **Evaluation – What was good and bad about the situation?** | When I think back to the situation I can see that <br><br> Something I have found out about myself is <br><br> I know I need to change the way I think about <br><br> It is important for me to |

| | |
|---|---|
| **Analysis – What sense can I make of the situation?** | I believe that _____<br><br>I still maintain that _____<br><br>I understand that if I had/hadn't _____<br><br>It would have been better if I had/hadn't _____<br><br>I agree that _____<br><br>I disagree that _____ |
| **Conclusion – What else could I have done?** | In conclusion I can see that _____<br><br>Upon reflection _____<br><br>I would never have thought about the situation in this way _____<br><br>The other thing I could have done was _____ |
| **Action plan – If it arose again what would I do?** | In the future I would like to _____<br><br>It is important to develop my thinking because _____<br><br>Moving forward I need to _____<br><br>If the situation arose again I would _____ |

## CASE STUDY
### Example of a reflection using Gibbs' framework

Martha, a second-year student nurse, reflects on an incident that occurred in her practice. She uses Gibbs' reflective cycle to guide her:

| | |
|---|---|
| **Description:** What happened? | In the morning I was assisting Rose, an elderly lady with dementia, with her personal hygiene. After chatting with Rose we agreed that she would like to have a shower. Physically, Rose is very independent but because of her dementia she needs prompting when carrying out activities like showering as she finds it difficult to carry them out in the correct sequence. Between us we gathered everything we would need and off we went to the bathroom. While Rose was undressing, I was reminding her what to do and how to work the shower. When Rose was in the shower, I realised that we had forgotten the shampoo. I was reluctant to leave Rose unsupervised in the shower; however, the ward was short-staffed that day and I did not want to press the call bell to ask someone else to get it. I told Rose to wait where she was while I left to go and fetch the shampoo from her locker. While I was gone Rose decided to get out of the shower. She tripped on the wet floor, fell and hurt her shoulder. |
| **Feelings:** What were you and/or others involved thinking and feeling? | Rose felt afraid and anxious while she was in the bathroom on her own. She was unsure what to do. When she fell getting out of the shower she was very upset and her shoulder was very sore. I felt guilty that Rose had fallen and that I had not cared for her properly and kept her safe.<br>Rose's family felt cross and disappointed with the care that Rose had received. They did not feel as confident as before about the nurses' ability to keep Rose safe. |

| | |
|---|---|
| **Evaluation:** What was good/bad and bad about the experience? | I had misjudged Rose's ability to understand and retain information. My preceptor was disappointed with me and said she now doubted my ability to take on responsibility. I had prioritised my embarrassment of having to admit to other staff members that I had forgotten the shampoo over Rose's safety. I feel way more embarrassed now about what happened subsequently. |
| **Analysis:** What sense can you make of the situation? | If I had planned and organised the shower with Rose better, I wouldn't have forgotten the shampoo in the first place. My inexperience with people who have dementia contributed to my bad judgment. I thought Rose would stay in the shower until I came back, as I was going to be really quick. |
| **Conclusion:** Sum up what could have been done | I have learned that, no matter what, I should always prioritise the safety of the person I am caring for. If I had planned the shower better I wouldn't have put Rose or myself in that situation. I have learned that the guilt I felt after Rose fell was far worse than any embarrassment I would have felt at pressing the call bell and asking another member of staff to get the shampoo. |
| **Action plan:** If a similar situation arose in the future, what would you do? | I need to pay more attention to planning when I am caring for people. If I am in a situation where I have made a mistake, I should never put a patient's safety at risk trying to cover it up. Patient safety will always be my priority from now on. |

## Exercise

Use Gibbs' reflective framework to reflect on an experience that you had in your work placement.

Share your reflections with your classmates – you will learn from hearing about each other's experiences.

Remember to protect the confidentiality of the people involved in the experience.

# Record-keeping and reporting

Record-keeping is an integral part of care. The basic principle in record-keeping is: 'If it has not been recorded, it has not been done.' Good record-keeping is an indicator of a skilled nurse. Nurses are accountable for their practice and good record-keeping and reporting practice allows them to document and provide evidence of their actions.

> According to the NMBI:
>
> The quality of records maintained by nurses and midwives is a reflection of the quality of the care provided by them to patients. Nurses and midwives are professionally and legally accountable and responsible for the standard of practice which they deliver and to which they contribute. Good practice in record management is an integral part of quality nursing and midwifery practice. (NMBI 2015a)

Maintaining good clinical records is essential for the following reasons:

1. To **document** nursing and midwifery care. At a minimum a patient record should include the following:
   * An accurate assessment of the person's physical, psychological and social wellbeing, and, whenever necessary, the views and observations of family members in relation to that assessment.
   * Evidence of decision-making and care delivery by nurses and midwives.
   * An evaluation of the effectiveness, or otherwise, of the nursing/midwifery care provided.
2. To **facilitate communication** between the patient, the family and all members of the healthcare team.
3. To **provide documentary evidence** of the delivery of quality patient care in relation to the following:
   * Nursing and midwifery decision-making
   * Continuity of care between health professionals including advice and instructions
   * Clinical audit
   * Debriefing of patients

* Dealing with complaints
* Fitness to practice enquiries
* Nursing/midwifery legal enquiries
* Teaching nursing and midwifery students
* Reflecting on and evaluating practice
* Research of nursing and midwifery practice – subject to ethical considerations.

## CONFIDENTIALITY

People have a right to expect that their personal information remains private. The nurse's role in safeguarding confidentiality extends to all forms of record management, including the appropriate use of technology. Nurses have a duty to familiarise themselves with the relevant policies in their place of employment, in relation to record management and electronic access.

## RULES FOR GOOD RECORD-KEEPING

* Use a black pen for handwritten records; never use pencil.
* When recording time and date, use the 24-hour clock.
* Record factual, objective details, rather than opinions. For example, rather than 'Anne Jones was drunk', record: 'Anne Jones had a smell of alcohol on her breath, her gait was unsteady and her speech was slurred.'
* When recording clinical practice, the person's name and record number must be on every page.
* Record events in chronological order.
* If an error is made in the records, put a bracket around it and draw a single line through it, and sign and date the error.
* Use your full signature always, unless the document specifies that initials are to be used.
* Do not alter what has already been written or use erasure fluid.

## RECORDING CLINICAL PRACTICE

When recording clinical practice, accuracy and clarity are essential. Examples of clinical practice might be the administration of medicines, the measuring of physiological observations or carrying out a procedure, e.g. inserting a urinary catheter or an intravenous cannula.

We will revisit this aspect of the nurse's role in Chapters 10 and 12 and you will learn how to ensure that recordings are accurate and clear.

## REPORTING

Nurses work in teams with other nurses and with healthcare professionals from other disciplines. For the benefit of the patient, it is important to share relevant information among healthcare professionals.

> Reports are made:
>
> Immediately – Thoroughly – Accurately

Use a notepad and pen to write down information for recording. Report only facts, not opinions. Report what you observed yourself or know for a fact, not what someone else said or what you expect to happen.

> ### DEFINITIONS
>
> **Objective** data is what is observed using the senses.
>
> **Subjective** data is what is told to the nurse by another party, e.g. a family member.

Reporting can be either oral or written.

When writing a report:

* use short, concise phrases
* always record information after care has been provided
* make sure writing is legible and neat
* record in a logical and chronological order
* use only accepted abbreviations
* avoid using words that have more than one meaning. (NMBI 2015a).

# REVISION QUESTIONS

1. Outline the difference between empathy and sympathy.
2. Outline some differences between personal relationships and therapeutic relationships.
3. Describe, in your own words, what you understand by the term 'advocacy'.
4. Give some examples of when a nurse might need to advocate on behalf of a patient or their family.
5. What is the purpose of reflection in nursing practice?
6. Explain why it is important for a nurse to be accurate when recording clinical practice.
7. Explain the difference between objective and subjective data when writing reports in relation to patient care.

# People Moving and Handling

In this chapter you will learn about:

* Manual handling/people moving and handling practices in healthcare
* How the body works in relation to manual handling
* Anatomy and biomechanics regarding manual handling injuries to the back
* Legislation on manual handling
* Risk assessment and communication

## Introduction

The general view of manual handling/patient moving and handling training in the healthcare workplace is at best resignation and at worst antipathy. If you are ever brave enough to suggest manual handling/people moving and handling training to healthcare staff you will probably get responses like 'Do I really have to do it again?', 'It's a complete waste of time' or 'Actually, I am rather tired, so I can have a snooze during the class.' This attitude prevails despite the fact that manual handling and people moving and handling are an integral part of the day-to-day work of healthcare staff. Every day healthcare staff assist people to stand, walk, get into and out of bed, assist them in the bathroom, help them to dress and generally support them in their activities of daily living; and healthcare staff use a wide range of equipment including hoists, wheelchairs, walking frames and sliding sheets.

Understanding the principles of manual handling/people moving and handling can ensure that all these activities are carried out with the minimum of risk to both healthcare staff and the people they are assisting.

Adopting a **positive approach** to manual handling/people moving and handling can transform an activity into an enabling and empowering experience for the person. Adopting a **negative approach** can reduce the activity to one of just moving the person from one location to another.

Healthcare staff who use the correct techniques, coupled with active and ongoing risk assessments, provide the person with the framework to move and be active with confidence. Standing up and moving around may appear insignificant to those who can do this freely but may be a major achievement for those who struggle with their mobility. Assisting people to achieve their potential in whatever form that may take should be considered both an honour and a privilege.

The first section of this chapter covers manual handling and how the body works in relation to manual handling. It includes anatomy and biomechanics with regard to manual handling injuries to the back, which is the most injured part of the body in workplace accidents, comprising 20 per cent of non-fatal injuries reported to the Health and Safety Authority (HSA 2020). This section will also include the legislation that relates to manual handling.

The second section covers people moving and handling and how to apply manual handling techniques when assisting people to mobilise. This will include risk assessment, communication and people handling techniques.

# Manual handling

### DEFINITION

The HSA defines **manual handling** as: 'Any transporting or supporting of a load by one or more employees and including lifting, putting down, pushing, carrying or moving a load which … involves risks particularly of back injury to employees' (HSA 2007).

### Top five reported non-fatal injuries by trigger, 2019, and five-year average 2015–2019 (HSA)

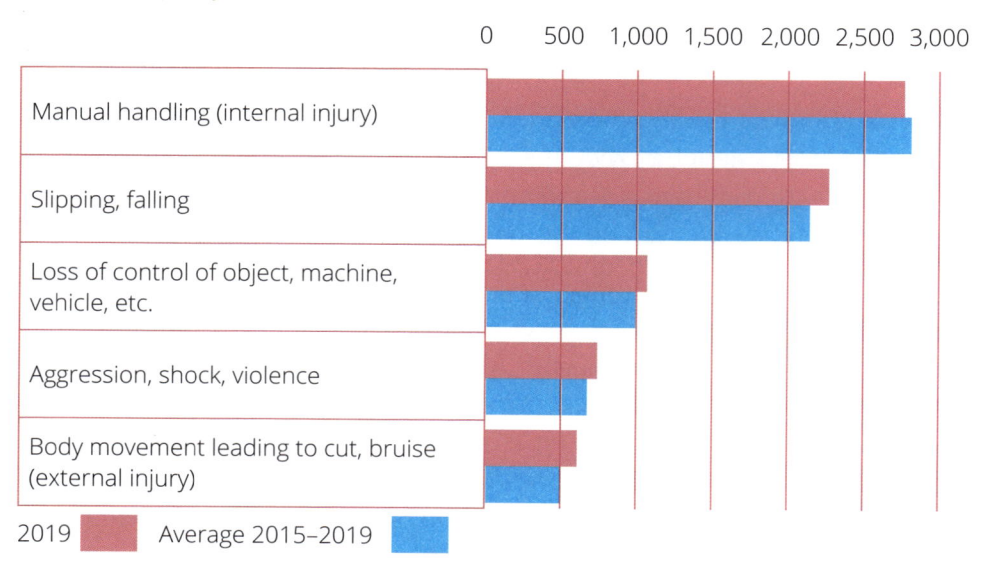

|  | |
|---|---|
| Manual handling (internal injury) | ~2700 (2019) / ~2800 (Avg) |
| Slipping, falling | ~2200 / ~2000 |
| Loss of control of object, machine, vehicle, etc. | ~750 / ~600 |
| Aggression, shock, violence | ~500 / ~450 |
| Body movement leading to cut, bruise (external injury) | ~450 / ~400 |

■ 2019   ■ Average 2015–2019

The importance of correct manual handling practices is highlighted by the HSA in its annual review of workplace injuries 2018–2019. The statistics identify manual handling (internal injuries) as the most common workplace injury.

This is also reflected in the statistics for the health and social care sector.

### Top three reported non-fatal triggers in health and social work, 2019 (HSA)

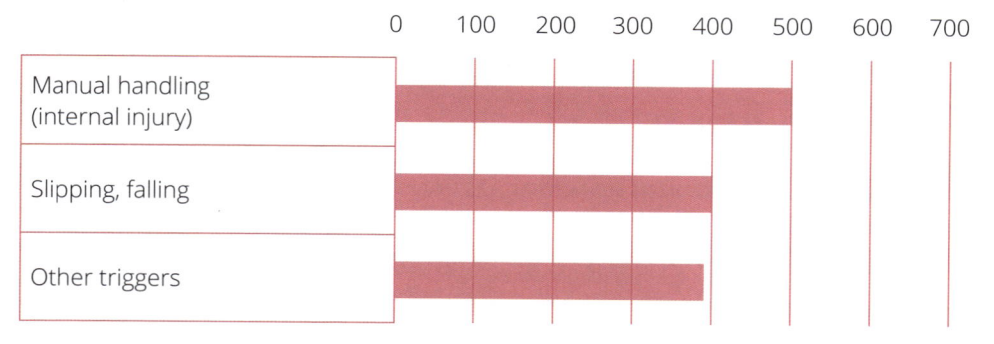

|  | |
|---|---|
| Manual handling (internal injury) | ~550 |
| Slipping, falling | ~450 |
| Other triggers | ~400 |

### Other important statistics

* Fifty per cent of all occupational illnesses relate to musculoskeletal ill health.
* Twenty-four per cent of all injuries are to the back.
* Between 60 and 90 per cent of people will suffer from some type of low back injury during their working life.

* Forty-two per cent of people are suffering at any one time.
* Sixty per cent will recover within six weeks.
* Between 20 and 40 per cent will have a recurrence. (HSA 2015)

# Anatomy

Anatomy is the scientific study of the structure of the body. It is important to have knowledge of the basic tenets of anatomy in order to understand and apply effective manual handling/people moving techniques. The key areas to consider are the spine, the skeletal muscles, tendons, ligaments and nerves.

## THE SPINE

Also called the vertebral column, backbone or spinal column, the spine consists of a series of bones called vertebrae. An adult spine typically contains twenty-six vertebrae, in different sections:

* Cervical (seven vertebrae)
* Thoracic (twelve vertebrae)
* Lumbar (five vertebrae)
* Sacrum (five fused vertebrae making one bone)
* Coccyx (four fused vertebrae making one bone).

When viewed from the front, the spine looks like a straight column, but from the side we can see that in fact it has four curves. This increases the strength of the spine, helps us to balance, allows the spine to absorb shock and helps to protect the vertebrae from fractures.

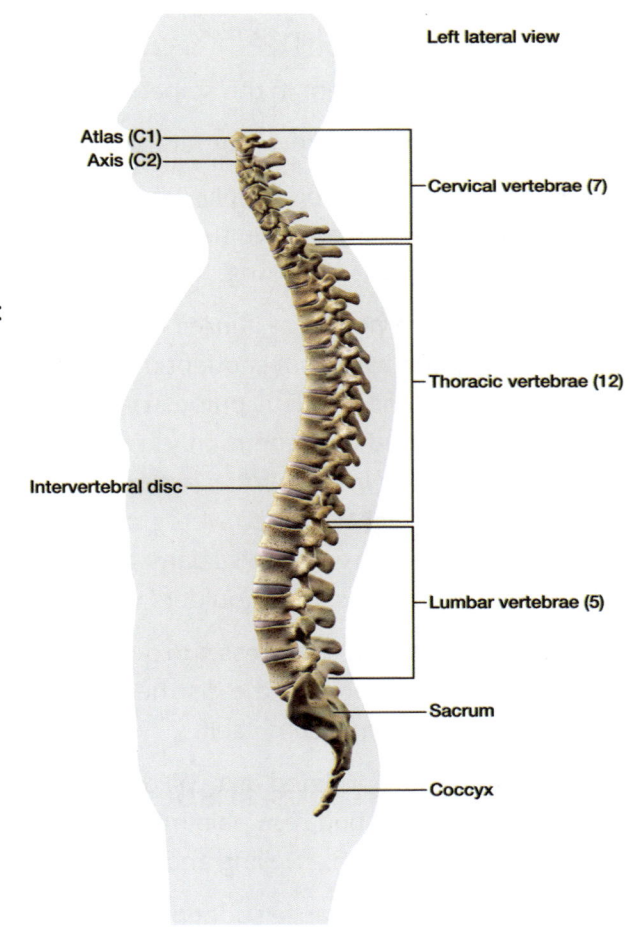

The spine performs various important functions:

* Protection of the spinal cord (part of the central nervous system)
* Support of the head
* Provision of attachment sites for the ribs, muscles, ligaments and tendons.

## INTERVERTEBRAL DISCS

These discs sit between each of the vertebrae in the spine. They have a fibrous outer layer called the annulus fibrosus, which protects the nucleus pulposus, a soft, toothpaste-like, elastic substance inside the disc. The purpose of the discs is to:

* form strong joints
* allow space for nerves
* enable movement in the spine
* absorb shock (vertical compression).

Discs have a poor blood supply, which means that they do not heal quickly. They also have a poor nerve supply, making it difficult to recognise when damage or injury is occurring.

If the spinal ligaments are injured or weakened, this can place extra pressure on the disc and cause subsequent damage and tearing to the annulus fibrosus. The inner nucleus pulposus may then protrude from the disc. This is called a herniated disc, commonly known as a slipped disc. Herniated discs occur most often in the lumbar area of the spine as this is where we bear much of our weight and also where we tend to flex and bend from. Care workers are also prone to disc damage in the cervical spine due to an over-reliance on the arms and shoulders when moving clients.

Herniated discs can compress surrounding nerves, causing pain, weakness and altered sensations. If the disc herniates posteriorly it can cause neuron damage to the spinal cord itself.

Treatment for a herniated disc will depend on the severity of the injury. Typical measures include bed rest, pain medication, physical therapy, injections to reduce inflammation, swelling and pressure, and surgery.

It is also possible to cause sudden major injury to the disc (a prolapsed disc). This is caused by twisting to the side, forward or back while carrying a load. In patient care it is often caused by sudden, unexpected movement of a patient when the carer is badly positioned.

## SKELETAL MUSCLES

Skeletal muscles consist of muscle fibres, connective tissue and a good supply of blood vessels and nerves. Muscles can contract and relax to facilitate movement in the body.

Muscle strain is a tearing of the muscle fibres or the tendon that attaches it to the bone. This can occur when the muscle is stretched beyond its limit. For healthcare workers this can happen when performing sudden, heavy lifting.

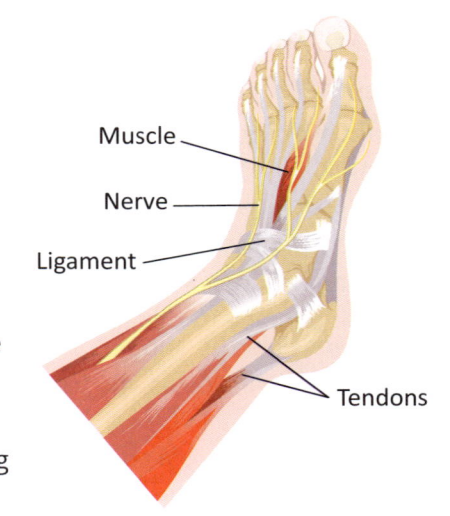

Repetitive strain injuries or muscular imbalances can also result from repeated movements, poor posture and poor biomechanics. Healthcare workers need to be mindful of this as they are often required to perform repetitive tasks with their clients, such as rolling and assisting from a sitting to standing position.

To avoid injury, carefully consider your body position so that you can make use of the stronger muscles in your body such as the glutes, hamstrings and quadriceps instead of placing excessive strain on your arm, shoulder and neck muscles or on your spine.

As we age, we all experience skeletal muscle loss. Between the ages of thirty and fifty, most people will lose approximately 10 per cent of their muscle mass and will experience a decrease in strength, slower reflexes and flexibility loss. Another 40 per cent is usually lost between the ages of fifty and eighty. Typically, the muscles in the lower limbs will weaken first, which means that elderly clients may find activities such as climbing stairs and getting up from a sitting position a greater challenge.

## TENDONS

A tendon is strong connective tissue that attaches a muscle to a bone. Overuse or overloading of tendons can lead to inflammation, called tendonitis. It can also contribute to the development of carpal tunnel syndrome. Healthcare workers should pay particular attention to the tendons in their hands as pinching actions to lift heavy limbs can lead to these conditions or to partial/full tendon ruptures (tears). Always use open palms ('soft hands') when moving clients.

## LIGAMENTS

Ligaments are fibre bundles that hold bones together in a joint. They allow flexibility and movement at the joint while preventing the bone from dislocating. If ligaments are damaged or overstretched, this can introduce greater flexibility into the joint, which will make it less structurally stable and more likely to dislocate. Ligaments also have poor blood supply, which delays the healing process. Repetitive straining activities and poor body positioning can cause damage to the ligaments.

## NERVES

The nervous system is a complex mechanism that allows us to gather and interpret information and to instruct the body to react accordingly. A healthy nervous system is vital to the correct functioning of our entire body. Damage, irritation or compression of the nerves can cause extreme pain and impaired bodily function. A common nervous injury is sciatica which is caused by compression or irritation of the sciatic nerve. Symptoms typically include pain and also possible loss of sensation or function.

(Tortora, Derrickson 2014)

# Biomechanics

Each person has a centre of gravity located, when standing up, in the navel region. The force of gravity runs from the centre of gravity downwards to the floor. We maintain balance when standing by keeping our centre of gravity directly above our base of support (our feet) and we can improve our balance by keeping a wide base of support (a wide stance). We usually stand still with our feet shoulder-width apart to ensure balance and stability.

A load held in front or to the sides, away from the body, disturbs the balance, and tension is generated in the back muscles to compensate, forming a lever effect. For an average person, holding a load at arm's length can impose up to ten times the stress experienced when holding the load close to the trunk of the body. Avoid generating excessive tension or strain on the back by holding loads close to the body.

When a person leans forward, the centre of gravity moves forward beyond the base of support and he/she becomes unstable. To counteract this, internal muscles, back ligaments and spinal discs are placed under pressure and other muscle groups are recruited, leading to tension and inefficient effort.

To make ourselves more stable we can increase the base of support by widening our stance, bending our knees to lower our centre of gravity, using an aid like a Zimmer frame or a crutch or by going on all fours.

The centre of gravity in a person lying flat is in the pelvis, so moving the pelvis will turn the body over. However, the centre of gravity of a person sitting in a bed is higher, making them more difficult to manoeuvre.

(Tortora, Derrickson 2014)

> To correctly move a load, whether it is a box or a body, we should have a wide stable base and keep that load close to the body.

# Legal rights and responsibilities

## DUTIES OF THE EMPLOYER

The employer must provide as follows:

- A safe place of work, including consideration of client behaviours; sanitary conditions; safe electrics; operative alarm systems
- Safe systems of work, including written care plans; appropriate equipment and staffing
- Safe access and exit, taking consideration of dangerous locations, particularly for single carers
- Safe plant and machinery: defective or incorrectly sized equipment must be repaired or replaced immediately
- Information: *full* client information including *current* medical status
- Instruction: phone assistance available at all times when working; supervisors visiting the site regularly
- Training: training of assistants.

## DUTIES OF THE EMPLOYEE

Employees must operate as follows:

- Comply with relevant safety and health laws
- Not be under the influence of an intoxicant (e.g. alcohol, strong over-the-counter medications)

- Not engage in improper conduct or behaviour, e.g. bullying and harassment
- Wear personal protective equipment (PPE) where necessary; know when to wear PPE and when not to
- Co-operate with the employer: follow the care plan and any client care instructions from a supervisor
- Not do anything that would place themselves or others at risk
- Report any problems, e.g. defective equipment; client behaviour or health issues; increasing infirmity; elder abuse suspicions.

# Safe lifting guidelines

**The procedure:**
- Assess the environment
- Assess the load
- Correct position of feet
- Load close to body
- Straight back
- Bend knees
- Correct grip
- Lift smoothly
- Do not twist.

**Assessing the environment:**
- Where is the load going?
- Are there obstructions in the way?
- Do you need to wedge doors open?
- Do you need to move furniture?
- Is there somewhere to set the load down, e.g. shower seat, garden seat, mobile seat, if there is doubt about client's stamina?

**Assessing the load:**

- How heavy is the load?
- Are there any sharp edges?
- Is the weight evenly distributed? (Keep the heaviest side nearest to your body.)
- What is the best way to hold the load?

**Lifting safely:**

- Lift the head up, straighten the back and look ahead before lifting.
- Place feet flat on the ground, comfortably apart, close to the load and in the direction you are going.
- Lower the body by relaxing the knees.
- Maintain a straight back (but not necessarily vertical).
- Keep the load close to your body.

**One-arm loads:**

- Lifting with one arm is best avoided.
- If unavoidable, keep the shoulders level and switch arms regularly. Do you or the client need a belt as additional support?

**Two-person lift:**

- Designate a lead carer to give the instructions. The other carer remains silent to avoid confusion.
- Your employer should try, where possible, to pair carers of a similar height to avoid injury to the taller carer, which may occur as a result of stooping.

**Awkward objects:**

- Stand at one corner with feet comfortably apart.
- Grasp the bottom inside and top outside corner.

**Lowering from a high place:**

- Check the weight and stability of the load.
- Check there is nothing on top of the load.
- Stand as close as possible to the load.
- Stand with feet apart, one foot in front of the other, legs flexed.

* Grip firmly and slide the object down your body.
* If possible, use a mechanical aid or get help.

**Lifting to a high place:**

* Avoid where possible.
* Lighten the load by dividing it into smaller loads.
* Make sure you are standing on a stable surface.
* Keep the load close to your body.
* Use a mechanical aid or get help if necessary.

# People moving and handling: the principles

(See the next chapter for moving and handling techniques.)

People moving and handling is about helping people who have difficulty with mobility. This can range from very little, such as a gentle hand when getting out of a chair, to complete dependence where the person needs assistance with all activities of daily living. The most important thing to remember is that the level of assistance should meet the requirements of the person. We help people where help is needed but we do not do things for people that they can do themselves – by doing this we actively disable them and encourage dependencies. Healthcare staff sometimes assist people when it is not necessary, and there are a number of reasons for this: staff are concerned for the welfare of the person and the possibility that they may fall and suffer an injury; staff have developed the habit of helping – they help one person, so they help every person regardless of their abilities; or time pressure to complete tasks means that it is easier and quicker to assist the person rather than letting them do it, which will take up too much time. The person should always be encouraged to keep themselves active and mobile and do as much for themselves as possible.

The following are the guidelines for people moving and handling for healthcare staff working in healthcare settings including hospitals, residential nursing homes and homecare.

> **Remember!**
> - Being dependent on others for basic care and mobility places a person in an extremely vulnerable position.
> - Always remember that it is a person you are moving, and they need to be treated gently and with respect.
> - Lack of mobility does not affect a person's right to choose how they live; the role of healthcare staff is to assist them to do this as far as is practically possible.
> - While ensuring the safety of the person, we should seek to maximise their independence and their ability to self-mobilise.

There are **four** building blocks in correct people moving and handling.

| Risk assessment | Communication | Manual handling techniques | Patient transfer techniques |

Ensuring the safety of **both** the person and the healthcare staff is the objective.

## RISK ASSESSMENT

We are all constantly risk-assessing the various situations in which we find ourselves to ascertain potential hazards for ourselves and those around us. However, with regard to people moving and handling, this needs to be more structured as the risk of injury can be high, depending on the mobility of the person. It is impossible to completely eliminate risks in people moving and handling as we are working with a wide range of people with mobility levels that are constantly changing for a variety of reasons. The person could be feeling unwell, could have difficulties understanding what we are trying to do, or, like us all at times, could just be having a bad day. Risk identification and management is a vital part of people moving and handling, and it is not a static situation.

The most important risk assessment is the one undertaken before you begin to move the person. Take the time to listen and talk with them as this will give you a good indication of how they are and whether they are ready or able to move.

A good approach is to remember that the person in front of you is your teacher and they are giving you the information and knowledge with which to work. We also need to remain alert to any changes in circumstances, particularly after a prolonged illness necessitating bed rest or a stay in hospital.

> By risk assessing at work, we identify hazards and risks, and this enables us to take preventive steps to minimise or eliminate those risks.

When carrying out the risk assessment, remember the acronym **TILE**:

**T**ask – What is the job that you have to do? Getting someone from sitting to standing? Moving a client from a bedroom to a shower?

**I**ndividual – your capabilities for carrying out the task with or without additional aids or support.

**L**oad – In patient care this is the patient or client – think about size, weight, height, physical and mental state.

**E**nvironment – the location of the action, the equipment available, the obstacles (furniture, floor coverings, door saddles and steps).

> ### T is for Task
> What are you trying to do? (For example, sit a person up in bed; hoist a person out of a chair; change sheets or bed clothing)

Does the job involve:

* holding loads away from the body, twisting, stooping, reaching upwards or awkward postures?
* long travel distances where you or the person could tire?
* forceful exertions (including lifting, pushing, pulling)?
* unpredictable movement of the load due to behavioural issues, medication effects, fatigue or changing blood pressure due to excessive sitting/lying?
* repetitive chores, e.g. repeatedly correcting the sitting position of the client?
* insufficient rest or recovery time?
* stressful/rushed work rate imposed by the process?

If you answer 'Yes' to any of the above, you have identified a risk!

Something needs to be done to eliminate or, at least, minimise that risk. This may involve additional assistance or the use of handling aids (belts, one-way slide, standing hoist) or it may simply require adjustment of the time allocated to the task.

* **Have a plan – be clear in your head what it is you are trying to achieve.** If the objective is to get the person up and out of bed in the morning, into the bathroom for a shower/bath, dressed and then to give them their breakfast, this can appear like a lot of work. Think it through before you start in order to eliminate or manage risks. In people moving and handling everything should be in place before you start assisting the person to move. If you are helping somebody who is unsteady on their feet to move from the bedroom to the bathroom, you do not want to end up in front of a closed bathroom door. The risk of an injury increases as you try to help them to remain stable and open the door at the same time.

* **Break down the overall objective into smaller tasks.** Concentrate on each task, one at a time, taking a small break in between to give both yourself and the person time to relax and let go of any build-up of stress. Concentrate initially on just getting the person to a sitting position in the bed, take a small break and then move on to the next task.

* **Have any necessary equipment ready.** If there is any equipment that you need you should have it ready **before** you start. For example, if you are sitting somebody up in bed and they may need the support of pillows when they are sitting, have the pillows at hand, ready to put into position immediately. If you need to transfer them to a wheelchair, have it ready by the side of the bed so they are not left sitting on the side of the bed for an extended period while you fetch it. If you need a support belt to assist them into a standing position, have it ready to put on them.

## I is for Individual (healthcare staff)

Think about:

* **Physical condition –** Do you have any reservations about your strength, agility and general physical ability to cope with the client/patient?

* **Illness –** Is there a risk of transferring infection to your client?

- **Pregnancy –** Are your current tasks safe to perform?
- **Training –** Are you sufficiently trained, e.g. in infection control, elder abuse, aggressive behaviour, dementia?

Where family members are directly involved in the care of the client, manual handling/patient moving and handling and other relevant training should also apply to them.

All healthcare staff should be frank and open with the supervisor/provider about any doubts or concerns they might have about caring for any particular client/patient.

**Are you, or the staff assisting you, physically capable of carrying out what you are proposing to do?** There are certain tasks that you may not be physically capable of carrying out and proper risk assessment takes this into account and comes up with an alternative solution.

**Are you, or the staff assisting you, up to the task on any given day?** If one or other is carrying an injury or is on medication that will impair their ability to carry out the task successfully, that should be looked at before the task is started.

Be absolutely sure that you have the physical capabilities to do what you are proposing to do. If there is any doubt, get help. Halfway through moving a person is too late to discover that you cannot manage it.

If the task requires two people, **do not attempt to do it by yourself** as you will place both yourself and the patient at a very high risk of injury.

> **Remember!**
> **Never take chances.**

## L is for Load (the person)

Is the person:
- heavy, bulky, tall, unwieldy or difficult to grasp?
- unstable?
- unpredictable?

The care plan should adequately address each of these issues and prescribe measures and equipment to cope with them. Where the healthcare staff judge these to be incorrect or inadequate, they should raise the matter with their supervisor.

Remember that under the Safety, Health and Welfare at Work Regulations 2007, the employer is obliged to mechanise, where possible, to minimise risk.

> **Remember!**
>
> You must **always** ask for permission before you put your hands on a client or patient.

Respect is a basic human right, so you must always ask the patient for their permission to touch them. This allows them to exercise their right to choose what happens to them and also gives them the opportunity to discuss any problems they may have with being moved or handled.

* **Eye contact:** Make eye contact with the person to explain what you are going to do. It will reassure the patient and it will also give you time to observe their current condition.
  - Are they tired and lethargic or alert and energised? Their condition and ability to assist will have a huge impact on how you help them to move.
  - Are they correctly dressed for the task? If they are expected to walk, they should have good secure footwear (not loose slippers or bedsocks). A satin nightdress may be too slippery to allow you to securely support the client while getting them to their feet or back into a chair.

* **Changing circumstances:** Remember that people change constantly and the person you are assisting is subject to change, the same as all of us.
  - Their mobility may vary at different times of the day depending on their energy levels.
  - Their mood may vary, which may have an effect on their willingness or ability to assist you.
  - There may be effects due to medication.
  - There may be understanding difficulties ranging from the complex area of dementia to the simple issue of not being able to hear clearly.

* **Physical size:** A client's physical size has a huge impact on moving and handling. If a person is very heavy or very tall, they are much more difficult to move. Moving a very heavy person in the bed can be successfully done by the use of **sliding sheets** as you are not lifting the person but sliding them on sheets designed to do this, which reduces the risk of skin friction for the patient and back injury for the healthcare staff.

## HOISTS

If a person is immobile and cannot weight-bear (stand upright on their feet taking their own weight), a **hoist** will be needed to move them. Using a hoist is not a high-risk operation if you follow the correct procedures. Before using a hoist, make sure to get training as there are areas that are of particular danger, such as using the incorrect sling type or size.

> **Remember!**
>
> You need two people to operate a hoist safely.

There is also a **sit-to-stand hoist** available for people who can weight-bear but cannot walk. This is used to transfer them from bed to chair, etc. without lifting them completely into the air. Again, these hoists are an extremely safe method of moving, but you need to be properly trained in their use.

The highest risk group are people who are mobile but unsteady. They must be encouraged to do as much as possible for themselves as this helps them retain whatever mobility they have. If they stop using their muscles, they will lose mobility very quickly.

There are various other moving and handling aids that are of great assistance. The **support belt** (or **gait belt**) is used for people who are unsteady on their feet. This is a very strong cushioned belt with handles which the person wears around their waist. The use of a support belt is strongly recommended for anybody who is unsteady on their feet as it gives both the person and their carer a greater sense of support and security. The **sit-to-stand or return belt** assists the person from sitting to standing and from standing to sitting. It is particularly useful for clients who are nervous and hesitant about standing because of a fear of falling.

Always remember that equipment should only be used when necessary and it is the role of the occupational therapist to assess the person and recommend equipment that may assist them to mobilise. It is a matter of assessing the individual needs of the person and coming up with a solution that is safe for everybody involved. If you see a change in the mobility of your patient, ask your supervisor to have the occupational therapist carry out a reassessment. Suggest a time when your client is having greatest difficulties (e.g. in the evening when they are tired).

## E is for Environment

Environmental issues to consider include as follows:

* **Constraints on posture**, e.g. lack of space – Should unnecessary furniture be removed or should beds or seats be repositioned?
* **Poor furniture** – Is a low chair leading to unnecessary dependency on the healthcare staff to assist? Are sofas too wide to allow access for the healthcare staff to the side?
* **Poor floors** – door saddles; external door draught excluders; tiles that are slippery when wet in showers/bathrooms/kitchens; very 'busy' patterned carpet, which can be confusing to dementia patients; highly polished wooden surfaces combined with bed socks.
* **Variations in levels** – small steps in corridors; steps outside external doors and in garden paths; difficulties reaching a bedroom upstairs on return from a period of hospitalisation.
* **Poor lighting conditions** – particularly difficult for dementia patients. Is there a need for automatic lighting at night activated by a pressure mat switch?
* **Hot/cold/wet/icy/humid conditions** – Is there a risk of overheating or hypothermia for you or your client? Is ice or rain making surfaces outside slippery for you or your client?
* **Strong air movement** – Is there a possibility that a strong draught will cause your client to fall?

Nursing homes and hospitals are purpose-built facilities with all the required equipment in rooms and corridors designed for their particular purpose. However, even here, poorly chosen furniture can lead to dependency by a client on the care staff. Chairs/seats should be of an appropriate height to facilitate independent movement by the client. Low, soft sofas and armchairs force a client to rely on care staff. Equally, slippery seating material can cause some clients to slump, necessitating repeated repositioning in the chair.

Most of our homes were not originally built to accommodate the specialised equipment needed for people with mobility difficulties. Carers often have to cope with small bedrooms and bathrooms that are unsuitable for somebody with mobility difficulties. While we must respect the right of the patient to arrange their home as they wish, we must also be aware that the safety of both the person and healthcare staff is vital. It may be necessary to make some changes in the arrangement of furniture (for instance moving a bed from a corner into the centre of a bedroom or relocating wardrobes, etc. to another room), but this must be discussed and agreed with the person and will require the involvement of your supervisor and the occupational therapist.

When a person returns home from a period in hospital, they may have lost considerable mobility due to long bed confinement. It is vital to reassess the environment at this point. Where previously the person used a first-floor bedroom, this may no longer be safe or practicable. Equally, door saddles, rugs, mats and draught excluders may now prove a challenge, particularly if the person is using a walking frame. This kind of reassessment may even be needed if a person has not spent a period in hospital but is simply losing mobility rapidly.

In people's homes there is also the added complication of personal items, pets, furniture and thick carpets, which make it impossible to move anything with wheels on it such as wheelchairs, walkers and hoists. Particular attention should be paid to floor coverings, steps, changes in floor levels, door saddles, slippery surfaces, narrow openings, etc.

The ideal situation is that healthcare staff can operate safely in the home environment with the least possible disruption to the patient. It is understandable that the person would prefer to not have to make changes to their living arrangements; however, it must be recognised that changes may have to be made. If things are having to be moved repeatedly to facilitate moving a person, this is an unnecessary strain on the healthcare staff and should be addressed.

Good communication is the key to reassuring the person that any changes that are being made are necessary and are for their own safety. Reducing the risk of a fall or injury ensures that the patient remains in their home, which is where they want to be.

> Under the Safety, Health and Welfare at Work Regulations 2007, the employer is obliged to assess risks and, where possible, eliminate, automate or mechanise to avoid injury to employees and others.

# Communication

Communication is vital for safe and effective patient moving and handling. Remember, communication is not just about speaking to the person; it includes body language, facial expressions and intonation. It is not necessarily what you say but how you say it that is most important, as this is what the person responds to.

If you are moving a person, it is of the utmost importance that they **understand clearly** what is about to take place and they are comfortable and confident with the procedure. People can become agitated when they do not understand what is happening and this can sometimes lead to responsive challenging behaviours.

**It is much easier to move a person if you have their co-operation and willingness to assist you in whatever way they can.**

Always **make eye contact** when speaking with the person – do not speak to the top of a person's head when they are sitting but make sure that you are **facing them** at the correct level and explain what is about to take place.

During any moving involving more than one healthcare staff there should be only one person giving the instructions. This reduces the risk of misunderstandings between carers and the person.

Good communication with supervisory staff is also vital so that they obtain the necessary equipment or get clients reassessed where necessary, provide assistance when difficulties arise and ensure sensible rostering.

## Manual handling techniques

The basic principles of manual handling **always** apply when you are moving a person:

* Stand (or kneel) as close as possible to what you are working on.
* Maintain a wide, stable base.
* Keep your head up and spine straight.
* Keep arms fully extended and relaxed.
* Use a soft palm grip.
* Point your feet in the direction you are going.

## People transfer techniques

* **Risk assess –** Carry out a risk assessment before you start.
* **Have a plan –** Plan in advance what you need to achieve.
* **Know the mobility levels of the person you are about to move** – Consult the care plan.
* **Communicate –** clearly and with both the person and co-workers.
* **Operate from the side rather than front –** This is less confrontational and encourages the person to actively participate. Avoid underarm lifting.
* **Be aware of your body –** Maintain correct body and foot position, keeping your head up, back straight and feet facing the direction you are going.
* **Use the appropriate equipment.**
* **Do not use equipment you are not trained to use.**
* **Maintain mobility –** Encourage the person to do as much as possible for themselves as it helps to maintain mobility.
* **Keep the person close –** This will reduce instability.
* **Seek assistance if necessary.**
* **Report any incidents immediately.**
* **Do not put yourself or anybody else at risk.**

## Remember!

Slow down – it's not a race!

# People Moving and Handling Techniques

In this chapter you will learn about:

* People moving and handling techniques to apply when assisting people to mobilise

## 1. Sit to stand

Think about your positioning at all times. Squat or sit instead of stooping to introduce yourself and give instructions. Take your time to risk assess. Remember, use face-to-face communication where possible. When giving instructions only one carer should speak. Respect your client's bodily integrity – inform them before there is any hands-on contact.

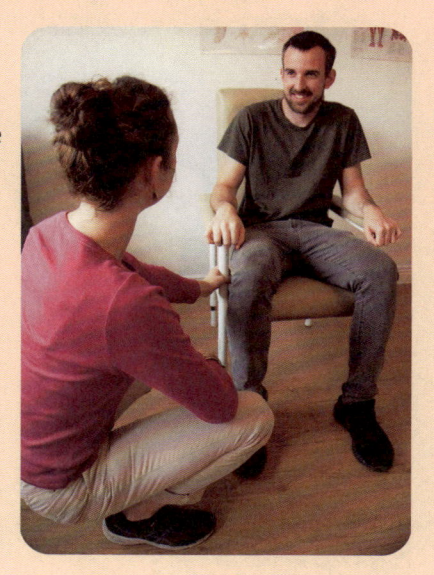

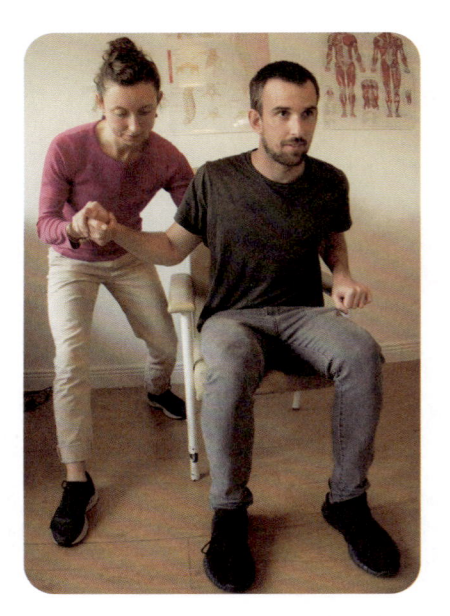

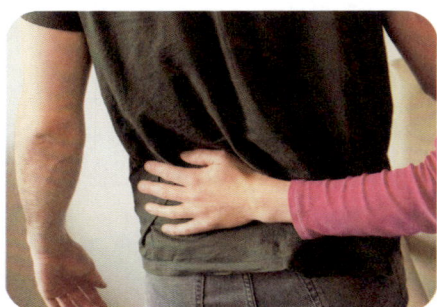

Remember to maintain a wide stable base. Stand close to the chair but give yourself some room to change position when you stand up. Position feet in the direction of travel.

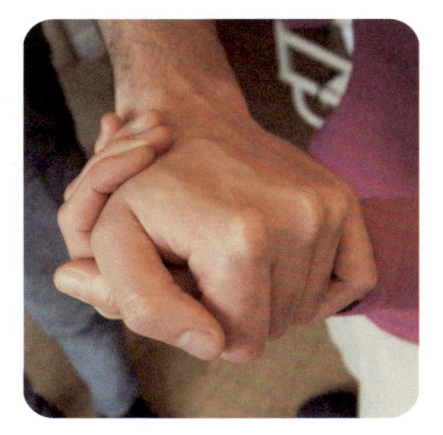

Do not interlock fingers or thumbs.

One hand should be placed on the client's pelvis for support.

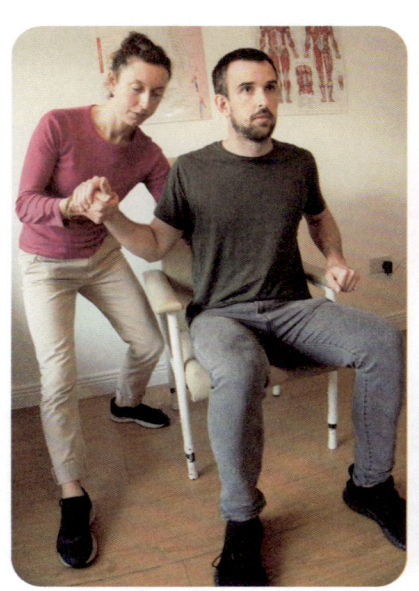

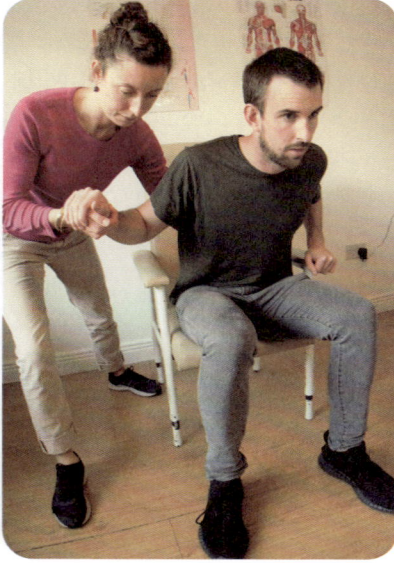

Rock back and forth to create momentum and to get the client's weight over their knees.

Change your foot position so that you are hip-to-hip with your client. Remain in this position until you are happy that they are stable.

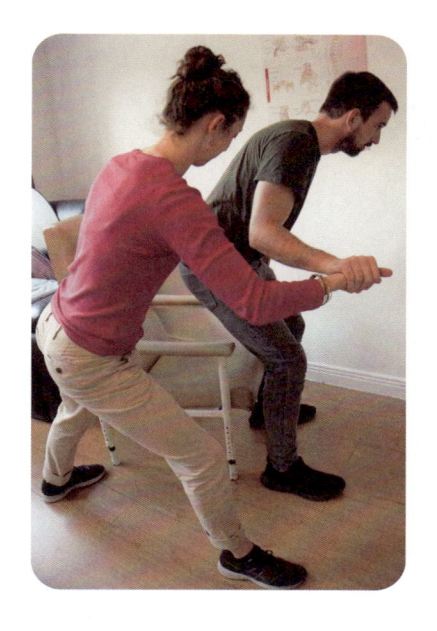

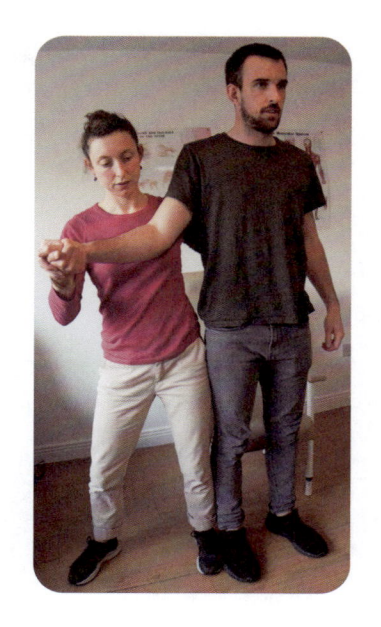

When assisting your client back into a chair, remember to adopt a wide stable base to maintain control and balance.

## 2. Rolling a client (roll and push)

### ROLL

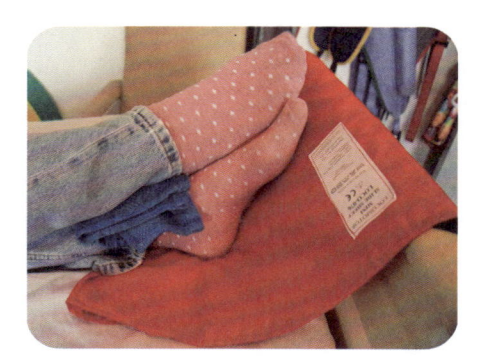

Before rolling the client, cross one ankle over the other – the top leg will be the leg furthest from the person performing the roll. Protect the client if they have delicate skin by using a small slide sheet under the heel and some padding between the legs.

Adopt a wide, stable base with both feet firmly on the floor. Keep your arms and back straight with your head up.

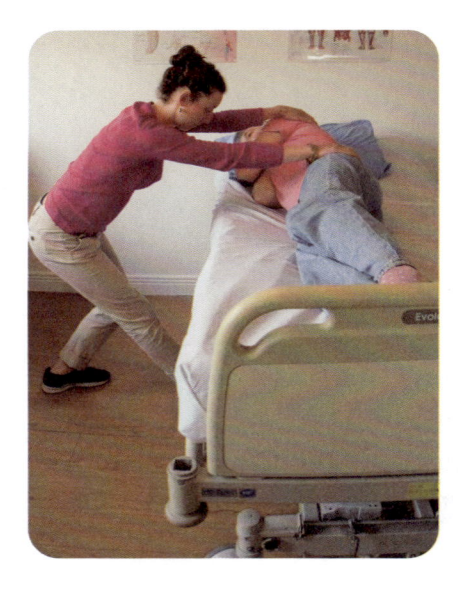

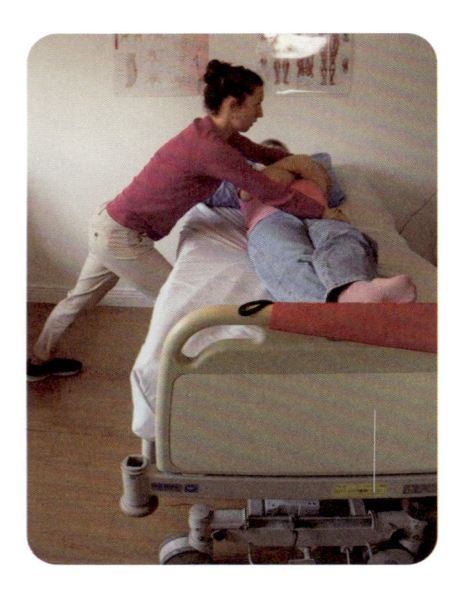

Roll back onto your back leg in a sitting motion. Make sure your back leg finishes bent.

Both feet remain on the floor. Arms and back remain straight and your head should be up.

Only stand in close to the client when you have finished the roll. Remain in this position to reassure the client while your colleague works on the opposite side.

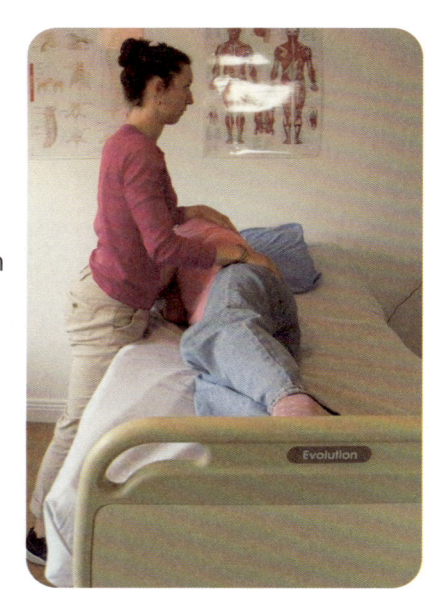

**PUSH**

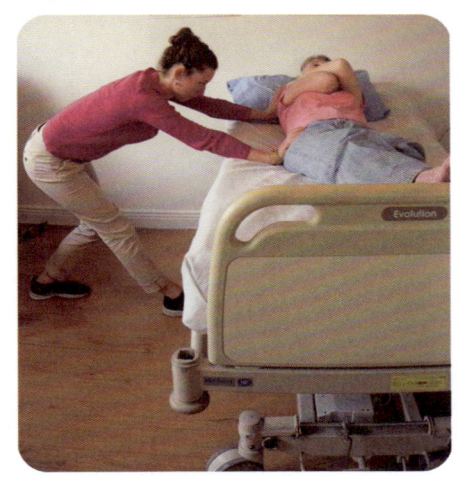

Start with your back leg bent, arms and back straight and head up.

Push up and forward, rolling your weight onto your front leg. You should finish with your front leg bent, arms and back straight and head up.

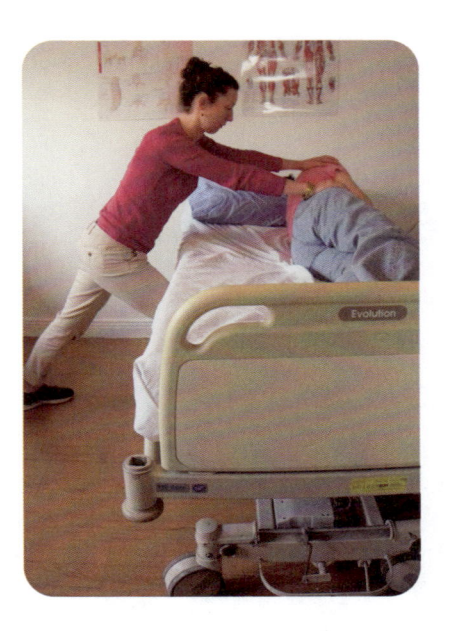

## 3. Slide sheets

Log roll the client and place the slide sheet flat on the bed behind them. Roll the sheet back on itself approximately halfway.

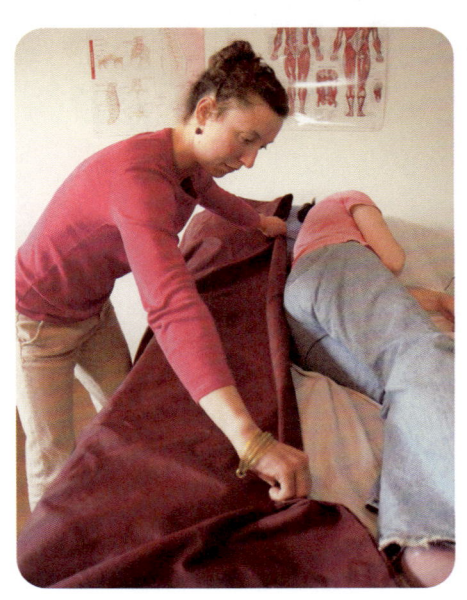

Push the sheet gently underneath the client. Concentrate on the light points of the body – ankles, knees, waist and neck.

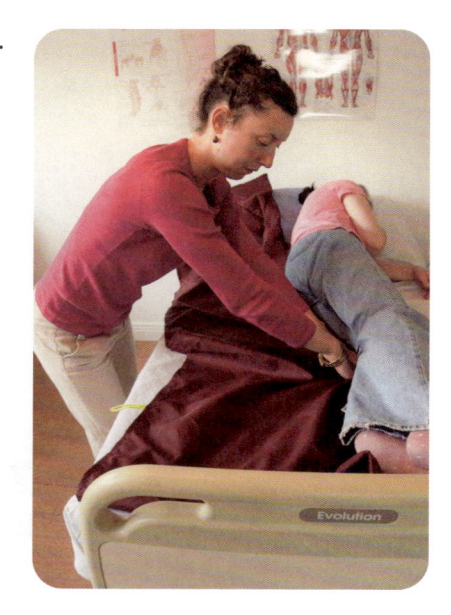

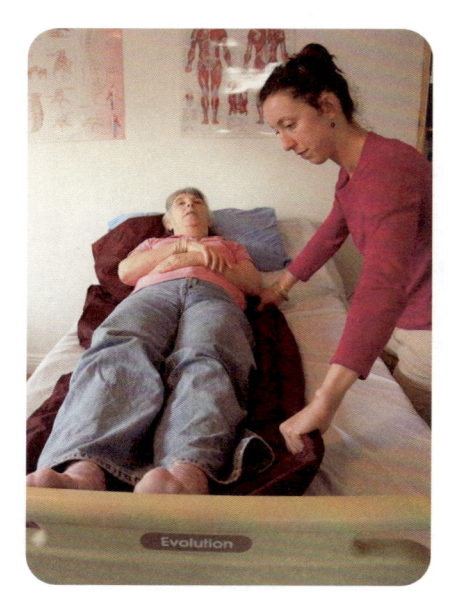

Roll the client onto their back and gently roll out the sheet from underneath them on the opposite side. Avoid a second roll to pull the sheet through.

To slide the client up the bed, both carers should adopt a wide, stable base at either side of the bed. Hold on to the top sheet only, with your knuckles pointing towards the ceiling. Remember to have your feet in the direction of travel and to keep your arms straight.

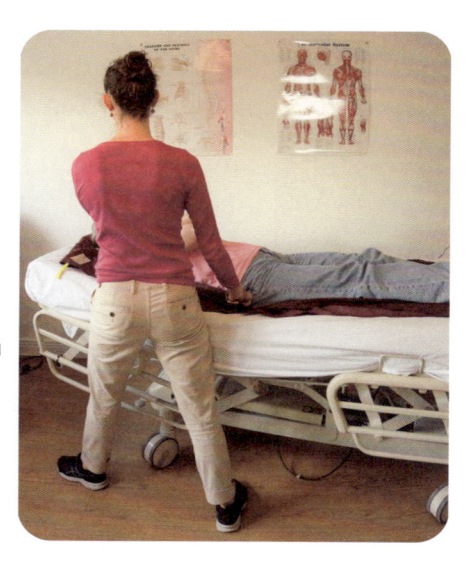

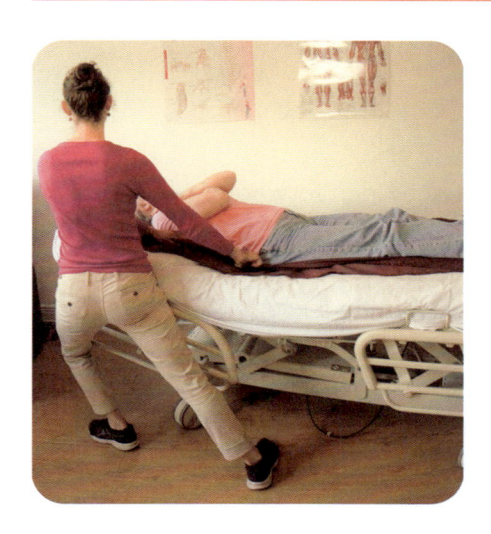

Finish with your front leg bent. Arms remain straight throughout. Do not bend your elbows. Remember to slide, not lift.

# 4. Hoisting

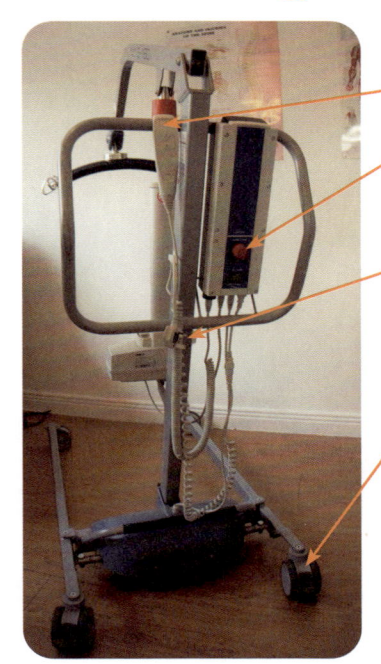

Remote control

On/Off button

Plug for charging (some hoists use a removable battery that can be placed in a separate re-charger)

Brakes. Do not apply the brakes when lifting and transferring to allow the hoist to centre over the client.

Hooks for attaching the sling

Emergency release

## Remember!

Hoisting requires two people and is a means of transfer, not transport.

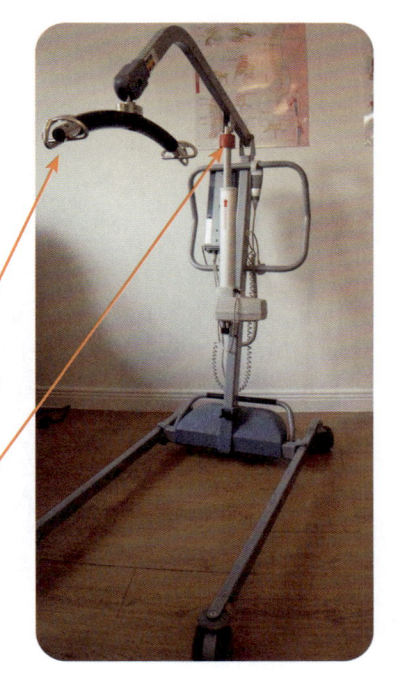

## 5. Raising a client

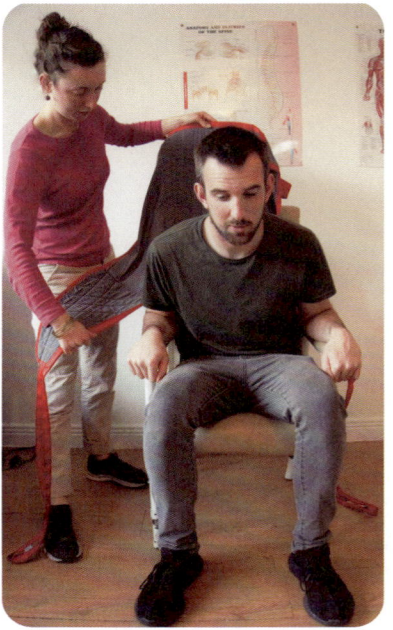

Ask the client to lean forward if they can. If they cannot do this it is possible to get the sling underneath them in a lying position using the roll technique (see page 95). Gently slide the sling behind the client.

The sling should be approximately shoulder height and level.

Squat in front of the client with your back straight and head up. Do not bend over from a standing position. Ensure the leg straps are tucked flat down the side of the client's legs and that both sides are level.

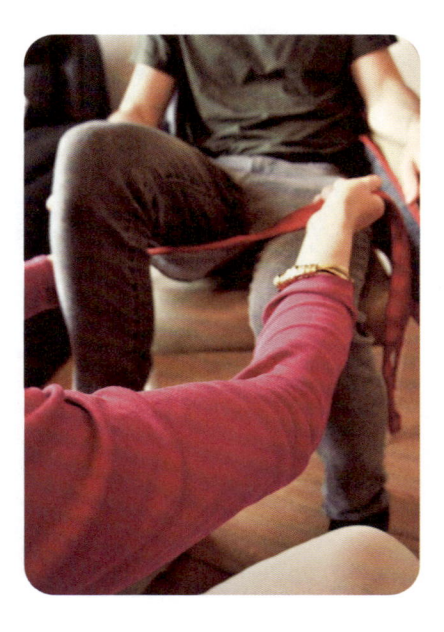

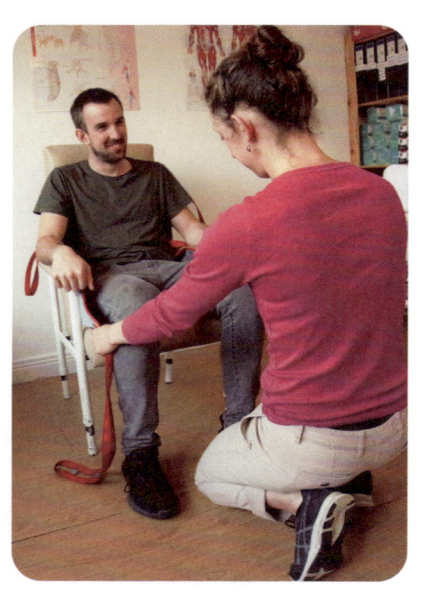

Prop one leg up on a footrest, footstool, box, your leg, etc., and pull the strap through underneath.

Make sure the strap is flat against the skin.

Cross the straps, one through the other, to prevent the legs drifting apart once they have been raised.

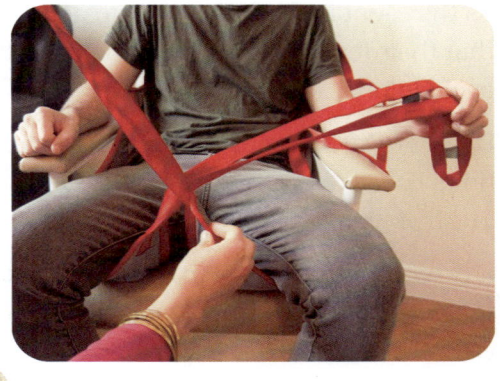

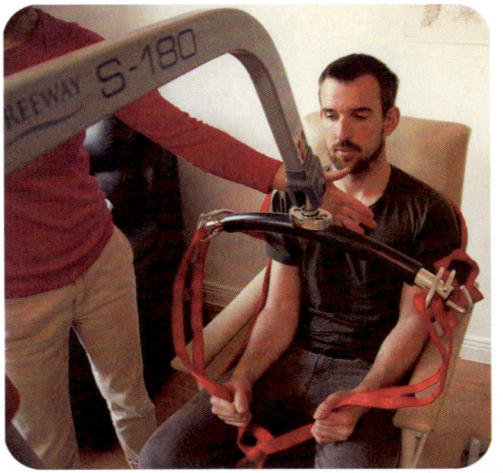

Attach the sling to the hoist. This may be by loops or clips. Make sure to check all straps to ensure they are correctly attached and matching either side.

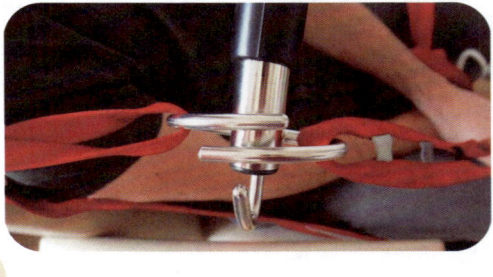

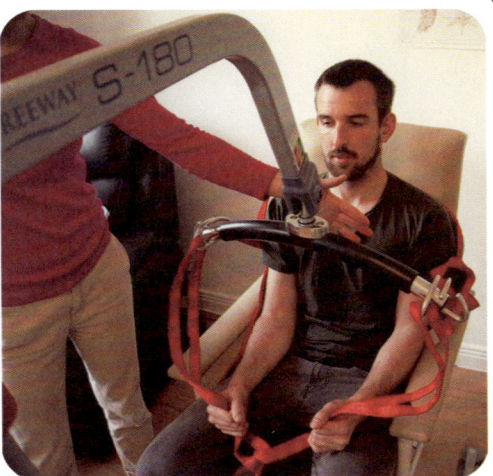

Top-down view of sling straps attached to the hoist

Protect the client's head from the bar when raising but do not stop the hoist moving in over their head.

PEOPLE MOVING AND HANDLING TECHNIQUES

101

As the client is raised, turn them gently so that their feet are away from the hoist to avoid injury.

Do not raise and move the hoist at the same time. Follow the procedure: Check, Raise, Check, Move.

A carer must remain with the client at all times to avoid swing. Only move the hoist when both carers are in position.

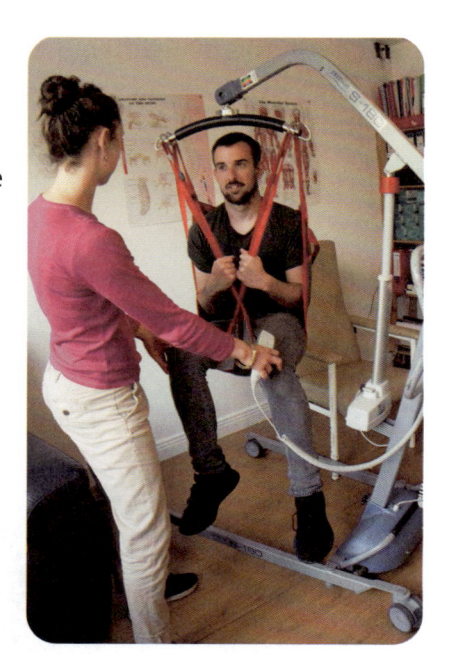

## 6. Repositioning a client

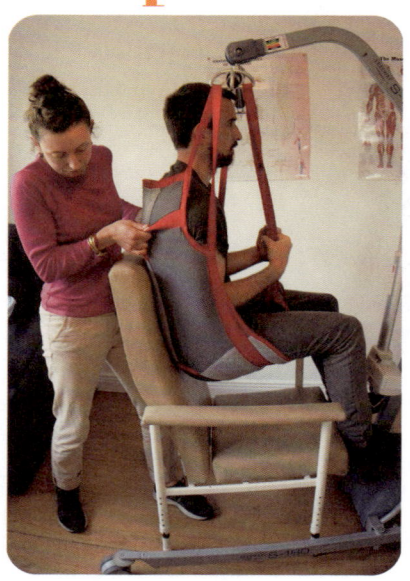

The carer should position themselves behind the chair, holding onto the straps at the back of the sling. Pull the client back into the chair as they are lowered to prevent slumping. A small amount of chair tilt is fine.

As the client makes contact with the chair, start to push the bar away from their face to avoid a head injury.

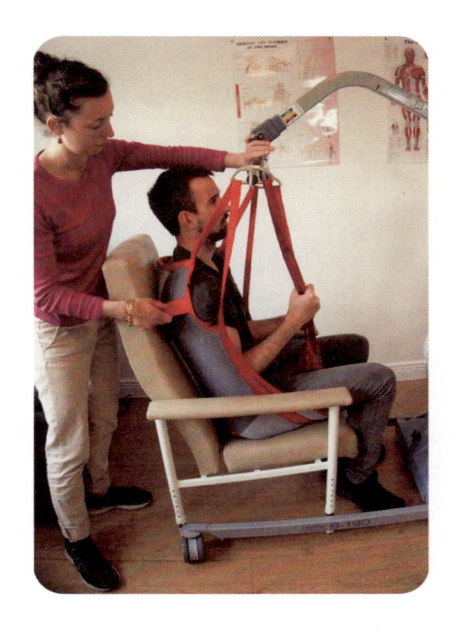

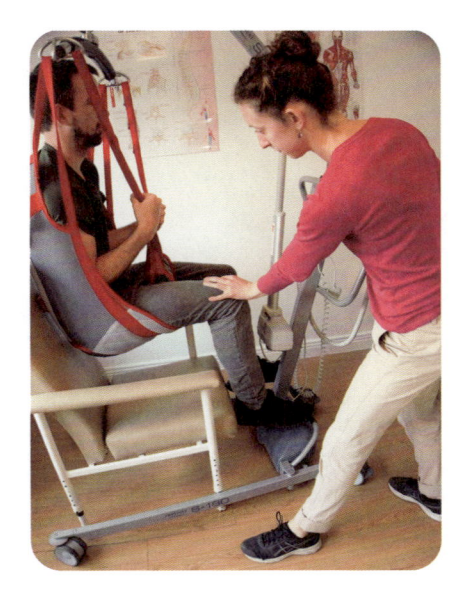

The carer operating the remote can assist to position the client correctly by gently pushing on their knee as they are lowered as long as that does not cause pain to or discomfort for the client.

# 7

# Infection Prevention and Control

In this chapter you will learn about:

* Infections
* The types of micro-organisms that cause infections
* The different ways in which micro-organisms spread
* The chain of infection
* Standard precautions

## Infections

Infections are diseases that make us unwell. Infections can affect our health and wellbeing and their effects can range from a mild to a severe illness and even death. Infections have always been a threat to good health and as a society we are continually striving to prevent them.

However, prevention is not always possible, so when infections do occur, we try to control them and to minimise their spread to others in the community.

# What is infection prevention and control?

> **DEFINITIONS**
>
> Infection **prevention** is the actions required to prevent an infectious micro-organism spreading from one person to another.
>
> Infection **control** is the actions required to contain the spread of an infection when it does occur.

Infections continue to challenge us, particularly infections caused by viruses. In our modern world, it seems that the more science discovers about infections, the more we need to know. Viruses can mutate and change and as soon as we have a vaccine or better treatments for the disease, another strain is identified, and we are back to where we started.

In our current pandemic, nurses have played a key role in the prevention and control of Covid-19 across the world. The principles that underpin nursing practice in the prevention and control of all infections remain the same as always, and the implementation of these practices has proved to be effective throughout the pandemic. It is where implementation has not been possible or has been compromised in some way that spread has occurred.

Although the scientific principles underpinning infection prevention and control are universal, the care that we provide varies from person to person, because every individual has different needs. The principles of person-centred care apply to nursing care in every context and situation. For example, if a person has an infection that causes diarrhoea, the nurse will need to wear disposable gloves and an apron when assisting them with toileting. This is universal – it will be the same for everyone. But each person receiving this care will feel differently about it. Being sensitive to this and providing the care and support that each individual requires is the essence of person-centred care.

Empathic care is required in every situation. When people who have recovered from infections reflect on how they felt while they were sick, they describe not only their physical symptoms but how they felt as a result of their illness. Accounts of fear, isolation, loneliness and sadness at not being able to see loved ones during their illness can be heartbreaking to listen to. These accounts remind nurses of the importance of taking steps to ensure their practice is empathic.

Reassurance, encouragement and acknowledgment of fear are important elements of empathic nursing care. Many barriers to this type of practice exist for nurses when caring for people with infections, the most challenging being the use of personal protective equipment (PPE). However, nurses are adaptable, and their professional values compel them to find ways of being caring and compassionate despite the barriers that exist for them and the people that they work with, and the care that they provide.

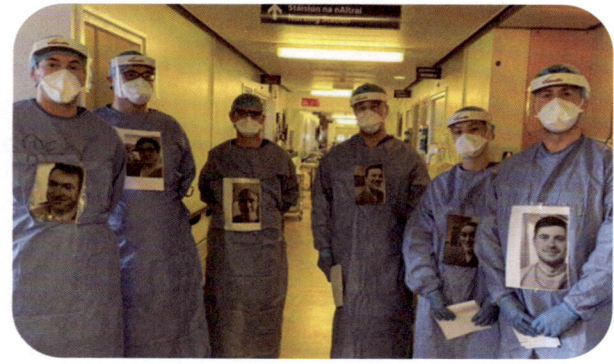

# Micro-organisms

Infectious diseases are caused by micro-organisms (microbes) that enter the body. Not all micro-organisms are harmful; the ones that cause disease are referred to as pathogenic.

Microbiology is the study of micro-organisms. Microbiologists play a key role in identifying pathogens and investigating how best to deal with them when they cause an infection.

There are four main types of pathogen that can cause infection in humans:

* Viruses
* Bacteria
* Fungi
* Parasites.

### TYPES OF MICRO-ORGANISM

#### VIRUSES

Viruses are tiny, non-cellular structures. They enter healthy cells within the body and damage or destroy them. They can be treated with anti-viral agents, if an anti-viral has been developed for that particular virus. Viruses can change their composition, and this can make the development of anti-viral drugs and preventive vaccines difficult.

**Antibiotics do not kill viruses.**

Diseases caused by viruses:

- Colds, seasonal influenza (e.g.H1N1) and respiratory tract infections, e.g. coronavirus
- Herpes, cold sores, warts
- Gastroenteritis, e.g. norovirus
- Viral meningitis
- Chicken pox, mumps, measles, rubella
- Hepatitis A, B and C
- Acquired immune deficiency syndrome (AIDS).

# BACTERIA

Bacteria are very small, single-celled organisms. Bacteria reproduce by dividing and multiplying. They can divide rapidly; a single bacterium could produce over a million bacteria in seven hours.

**Bacteria can be treated with antibiotics.**

Diseases caused by bacteria:

- Middle ear infection
- Impetigo
- Whooping cough
- Haemophilus influenzae type B (Hib)
- Diphtheria
- Tetanus
- Salmonella, shigellosis, gastroenteritis
- Meningitis
- Syphilis, gonorrhoea.

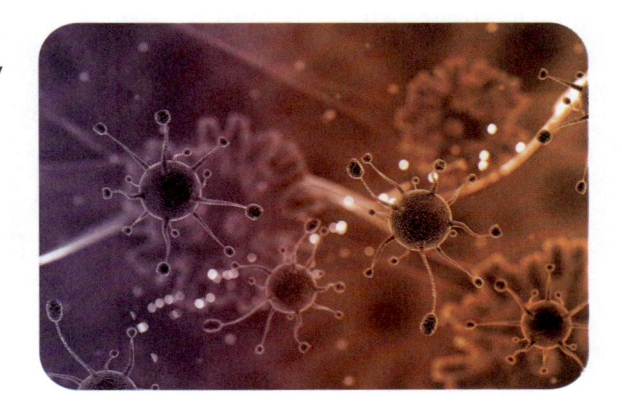

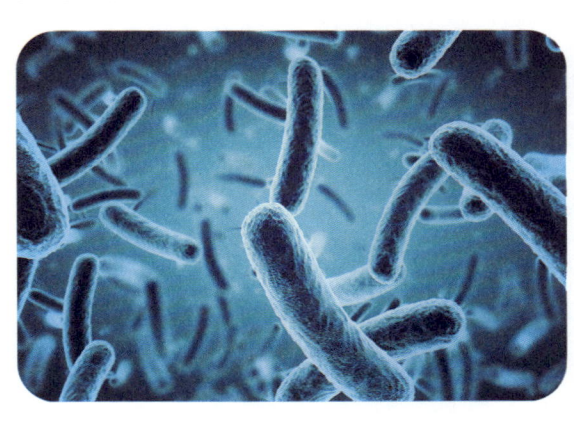

## FUNGI

Fungi include moulds, mildews, mushrooms and yeasts. Some are harmlessly present all the time in areas such as the mouth, skin, intestine and vagina and are prevented from multiplying by the presence of healthy bacteria. Fungi grow and cause infections of the skin and body linings, e.g. thrush, ringworm, athlete's foot.

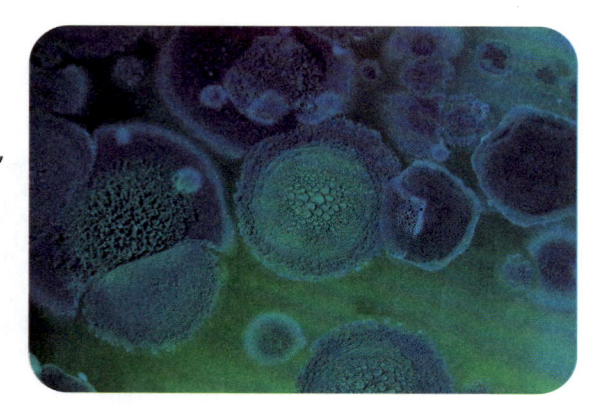

## PARASITES

Parasites are organisms that live in or on another living creature, referred to as the host. Parasites get into or onto the body to feed on healthy tissue, which causes tissue damage.

Parasites that cause infections include:

* mites, e.g. scabies, head lice
* metazoa, e.g. worms.

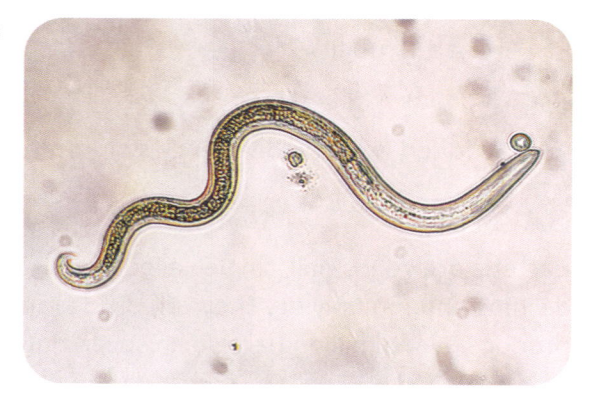

# Cross-infection

This is the term used for when a pathogenic micro-organism passes from one person to another. This can happen either directly or indirectly. Pathogens can survive outside the body in the air, on hands, on equipment and surfaces, in body fluids and in dust and dirt.

Micro-organisms will be present in any environment occupied by humans. The danger of introducing or transmitting infection when working in the healthcare environment must be recognised by nurses and other healthcare workers and steps taken to minimise this risk where possible.

## MODES OF TRANSMISSION

There are different ways in which pathogens can travel from their source to invade the body and cause illness. They can travel either directly or indirectly from one human to another.

> ### DEFINITIONS
>
> **Direct transmission –** Pathogens present in nasal secretions, when sneezed and suspended in the air, can be inhaled directly by another person, causing infection.
>
> **Indirect transmission –** Pathogens present in nasal secretions, when sneezed, may land on surfaces and be picked up on hands and thereby enter the mouth or nose of another person via unwashed hands, causing infection.

The four main modes of transmission are:

1. **Droplet or airborne infection**
   Pathogens spread when an infected person coughs, sneezes or breathes over another person. Nasal discharges and discharges from eyes, ears or throat are also very infectious. Dried-up discharges can be spread in the air and breathed in by others.

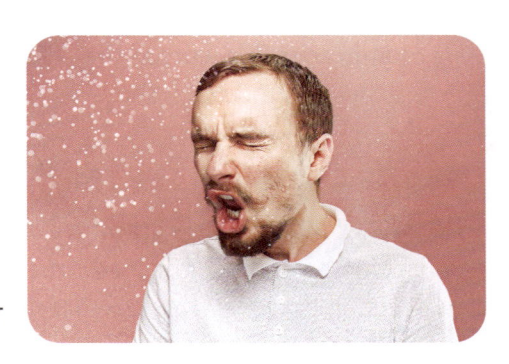

2. **Skin/direct contact**
   Infections are spread when the skin of an infected person comes into contact with the skin of another person. Cross-infection can also occur when skin comes into contact with contaminated surfaces, medical devices and equipment where pathogens are present.

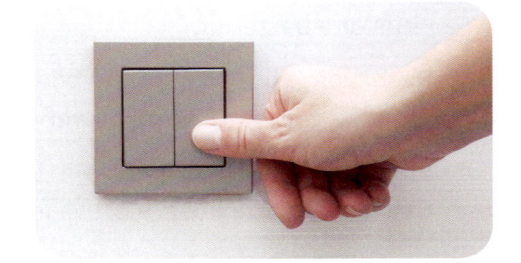

3. **Faecal–oral transmission**

    This usually occurs when hands become contaminated with faecal matter and infection can then spread to the mouth via the contaminated hands. This is a very common mode of transmission among young children, those with an intellectual disability and elderly people with a cognitive impairment. Spread can also happen via the objects that the person touches that are then touched by another person.

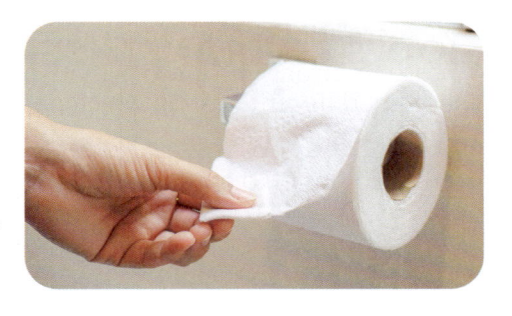

4. **Blood and bodily secretions**

    Some diseases are spread by blood-to-blood contact and by the bodily secretions of an infected person entering the bloodstream of another person through a break in the skin or via the mucous membranes, e.g. cuts in the skin or via the conjunctiva of the eyes.

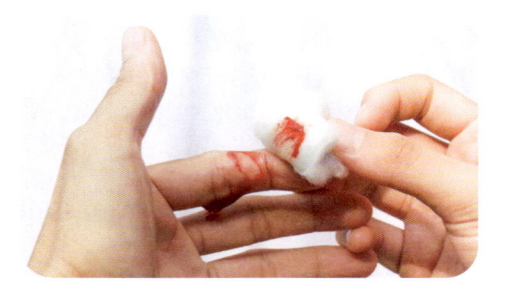

## CHAIN OF INFECTION

The chain of infection is a graphical representation of how cross-infection occurs. Nurses and healthcare workers must understand the chain of events that occur so that they can take precautions that will break the chain and prevent cross-infection from occurring.

* **Infectious agent** – the organism that causes the disease, commonly a virus or a bacterium

* **Reservoir** – the place in the body where the infectious agent lives and grows, e.g. mouth, nose, bowel, blood

* **Portal of exit** – any opening in the body that allows the infectious agent to leave, e.g. the nose, a break in the skin, the rectum

* **Means of transmission** – how the infectious agent travels from the infected person to another person, e.g. airborne, faecal–oral route, etc.

* **Portal of entry** – any opening that allows the infectious agent to enter the body, e.g. nose, mouth, break in the skin, urethra, etc.

* **Susceptible host** – a non-infected person who could become infected. It is important to be aware that some hosts may be more susceptible than others, depending on their immunity.

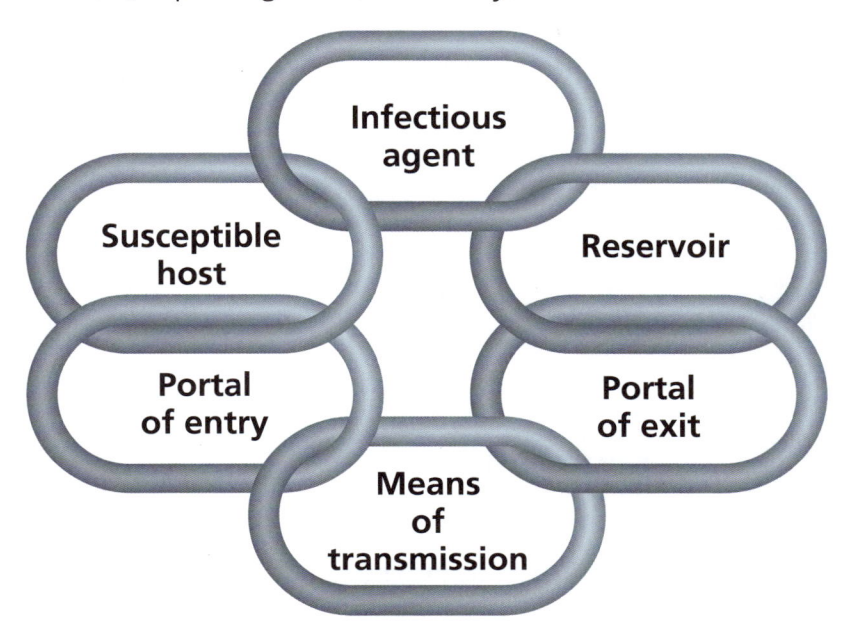

## Standard precautions

> ### DEFINITION
>
> **Standard precautions** are a range of practices that nurses and other healthcare workers can apply in their work setting. They are designed to reduce the risk of cross-infection (HSE 2009). Standard precautions are based on the principle that *all* blood, bodily fluids, secretions, excretions, broken skin and mucous membranes may contain pathogens.

The purpose of standard precautions is to break the chain of infection and therefore prevent a pathogen passing from one person to another (cross-infection).

Standard precautions include the following measures:

* Knowledge in the method and use of hand hygiene
* Correct use of PPE

- Respiratory etiquette
- Decontamination of patient equipment
- Safe management and disposal of waste
- Safe management of needlestick injuries
- Safe management of accidents and spillages
- Safe handling and management of linen and laundry
- Patient placement.

Standard precautions should be applied as standard principles by:

- **All** healthcare practitioners, for the care of
- **All** residents and patients
- **All** the time. (HSE 2017)

## HAND HYGIENE

Hand hygiene is widely acknowledged as the single most effective method of reducing the spread of micro-organisms in the healthcare environment. If it is performed effectively it contributes to both the eradication of micro-organisms and the prevention of the transmission of infection between clients, visitors and healthcare staff.

### FIVE MOMENTS OF HAND HYGIENE

The World Health Organization developed the 'Five Moments for Hand Hygiene', an approach that defines the key moments when healthcare workers should perform hand hygiene.

This approach recommends that healthcare workers clean their hands:

1. Before touching a patient
2. Before clean/aseptic procedure
3. After body fluid exposure risk
4. After touching a patient
5. After touching patient surroundings. (WHO 2006)

# SOCIAL HAND HYGIENE TECHNIQUE

The aim of handwashing is to remove dirt and organic material, dead skin and most transient organisms. This involves washing hands with plain liquid soap and warm water for at least fifteen seconds, then drying thoroughly with a disposable paper towel (HSE 2015b).

## Hand Hygiene Technique with Soap and Water

**Duration of the entire procedure:** 40-60 seconds

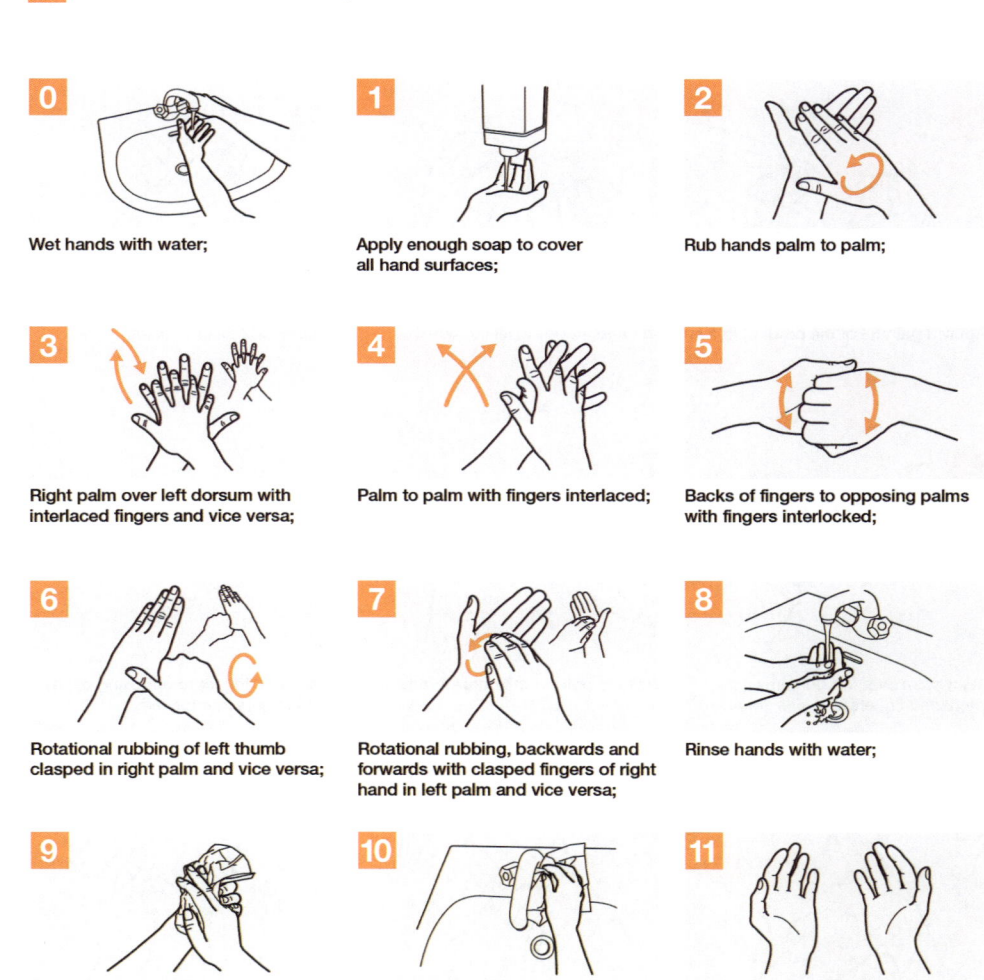

**0** Wet hands with water;

**1** Apply enough soap to cover all hand surfaces;

**2** Rub hands palm to palm;

**3** Right palm over left dorsum with interlaced fingers and vice versa;

**4** Palm to palm with fingers interlaced;

**5** Backs of fingers to opposing palms with fingers interlocked;

**6** Rotational rubbing of left thumb clasped in right palm and vice versa;

**7** Rotational rubbing, backwards and forwards with clasped fingers of right hand in left palm and vice versa;

**8** Rinse hands with water;

**9** Dry hands thoroughly with a single use towel;

**10** Use towel to turn off faucet;

**11** Your hands are now safe.

*Source: WHO Guidelines on Hand Hygiene in Health Care (2009)*

## ALCOHOL HAND RUB TECHNIQUE

Alcohol hand rubs can be used when hands are visibly clean. The hand rub solution must come into contact with all the surfaces of the hands and wrist. These products are very effective when applied to hands for a minimum of fifteen seconds. There is no need to dry hands afterwards as the solution will evaporate (HSE 2015b).

### Hand Hygiene Technique with Alcohol-Based Formulation

**Duration of the entire procedure:** 20-30 seconds

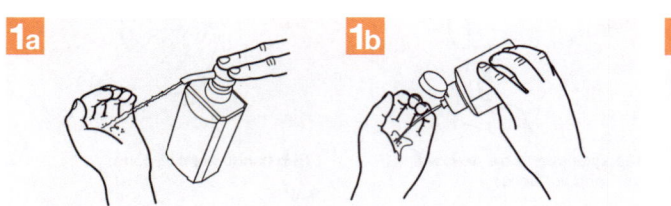

**1a / 1b** Apply a palmful of the product in a cupped hand, covering all surfaces;

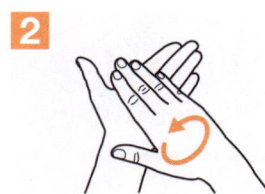

**2** Rub hands palm to palm;

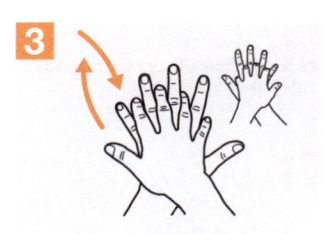

**3** Right palm over left dorsum with interlaced fingers and vice versa;

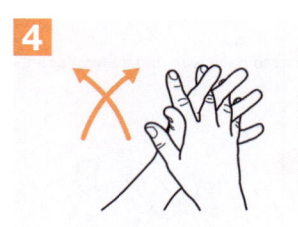

**4** Palm to palm with fingers interlaced;

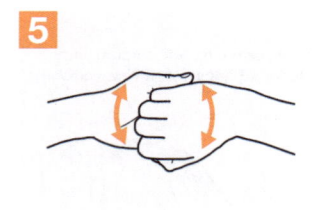

**5** Backs of fingers to opposing palms with fingers interlocked;

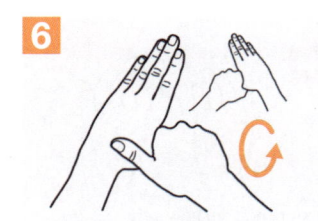

**6** Rotational rubbing of left thumb clasped in right palm and vice versa;

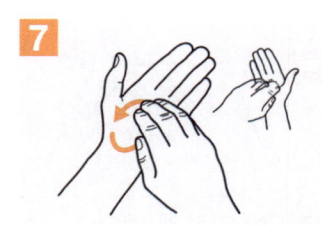

**7** Rotational rubbing, backwards and forwards with clasped fingers of right hand in left palm and vice versa;

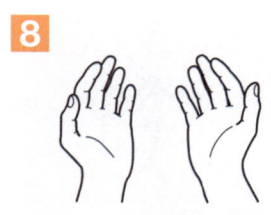

**8** Once dry, your hands are safe.

*Source: WHO Guidelines on Hand Hygiene in Health Care (2009)*

## PERSONAL PROTECTIVE EQUIPMENT AND CLOTHING

Personal protective equipment (PPE) and clothing may be worn when practising in clinical areas, residential care facilities or when working with clients requiring healthcare interventions in the community.

PPE consists of:

* gloves
* aprons/gowns
* face protection.

Remove PPE when the procedure is complete.

## DISPOSABLE GLOVES

Hand hygiene should always be carried out before and after donning gloves. Gloves should never be worn instead of carrying out hand hygiene.

Gloves should be:

* single-use items that conform to European Standards
* worn for all activities that carry a risk of exposure to blood, bodily fluids, secretions, excretions, sharps or contaminated instruments or patient equipment
* worn when touching mucous membranes and non-intact skin
* changed between caring for different clients/patients
* changed between different care episodes for the same client/patient
* sterile if contact anticipated with sterile body site.

Gloves are not needed when there is no possible risk of exposure to blood or body fluids or broken skin, e.g. assisting a client to wash, assisting with dressing or removing bed linen that is not soiled.

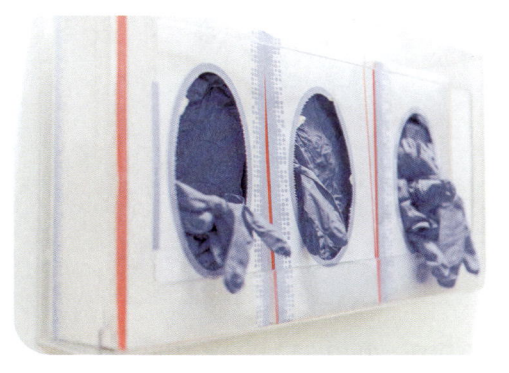

## DISPOSABLE APRONS

Disposable aprons should be worn where there is a risk that the front of the uniform/clothing may become exposed to blood, bodily fluids, secretions or excretions. If there is no risk, there is no need to wear an apron.

## PROTECTIVE GOWNS

For highly transmissible micro-organisms, e.g. coronavirus, it may be necessary to wear long-sleeved impervious gowns to prevent micro-organisms from contaminating the healthcare worker's skin or clothes.

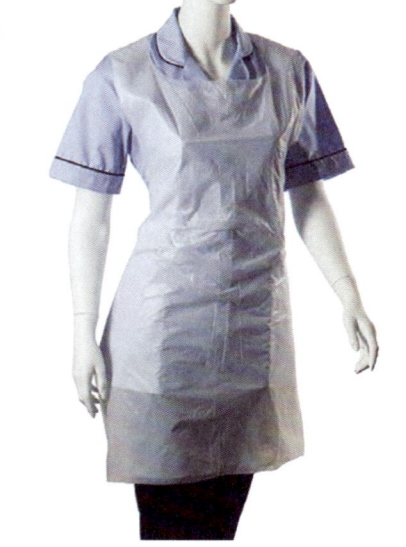

## FACE PROTECTION

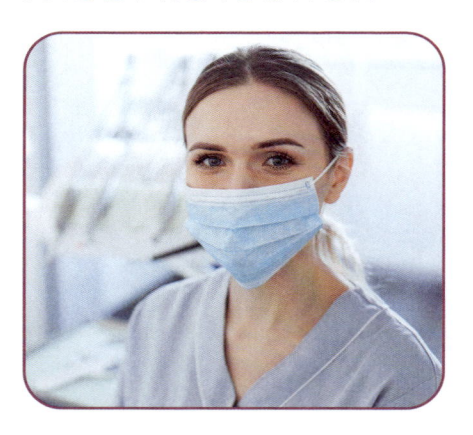

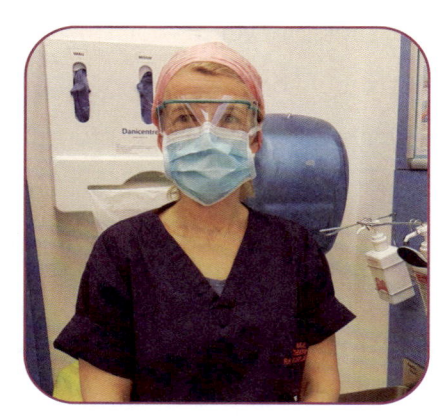

Face protection can be worn to protect the wearer from getting splashes to the face or eyes or to prevent the wearer from passing micro-organisms to a patient undergoing an invasive procedure.

Protection should be worn:

* when there is a risk of blood/bodily secretions/excretions splashing into the face or eyes
* when placing a catheter or injection into the spinal or epidural space or when assisting during a surgical procedure.

Face protection consists of one of the following:

* Face shield
* Fluid-repellent mask with separate goggles

* Fluid-repellent mask with eye shield
* Surgical masks, which prevent droplets from spreading from the wearer of the mask
* Masks with a high filtration rate, which protect the wearer from inhaling micro-organisms suspended in the air from the respiratory secretions of another person.

Face protection should be single-use or single-person use. Face shields and goggles can be reused by the same healthcare worker, *but* they must be adequately cleaned and disinfected between patients.

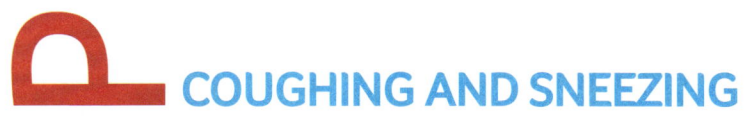

## RESPIRATORY PRECAUTIONS

### COVER UP

#### COUGHING AND SNEEZING

- Turn your head away from others
- Use a tissue to cover your nose and mouth

- Drop your tissue into a waste bin

- No tissues? Use your sleeve

- Clean your hands after discarding tissue using soap and water or alcohol gel for at least 15 seconds

These steps will help prevent the spread of colds, flu and other respiratory infections

*Courtesy of the HSE*

The aim of taking respiratory precautions is to prevent droplet and contact transmission of respiratory pathogens. This is especially important during seasonal outbreaks of viral respiratory tract infections, e.g. influenza, coronavirus.

As with all standard precautions, people who are infected, and members of the general public, play a key role in preventing infections spreading. Nurses should not only implement the precautions themselves but they also have a responsibility to educate others in relation to taking precautions. This is very important when trying to prevent the spread of respiratory infections in acute, residential and community settings.

Ensure adequate supplies of:

- tissues
- foot-operated waste bins
- hand hygiene facilities that are available in all departments, including waiting areas, throughout the facility.

Educate patients/visitors/carers on respiratory etiquette and cough hygiene using some, or all, of the following:

- Patient information leaflets
- Welcome packs
- Posters in all departments, especially waiting areas
- By example.

## DECONTAMINATION OF PATIENT EQUIPMENT

Decontamination is the combination of processes used to make an item safe for handling by staff and for further use.

There are three levels of decontamination:

- Cleaning
- Cleaning followed by disinfection
- Cleaning followed by sterilisation.

### CLEANING

This is a process that physically removes soiling, including large numbers of micro-organisms and the organic material on which they thrive. It does not destroy pathogens.

## DISINFECTION

Cleaning should always be carried out before disinfection. Disinfection is a process that reduces the number of micro-organisms. However, some pathogens will be resistant, e.g. bacterial spores. In hospitals disinfection is usually carried out using heat, e.g. bedpan washers. Chemical disinfection can also be carried out using a chlorine-based agent.

## STERILISATION

This is a physical or chemical process that completely destroys all micro-organisms including viruses and spores. Sterilisation involves using high temperatures, e.g. autoclaving surgical instruments (physical sterilisation), or using chemicals (chemical sterilisation) to destroy micro-organisms.

## SAFE MANAGEMENT OF WASTE

Healthcare waste is the solid or liquid waste arising from healthcare. The majority of healthcare waste generated in Ireland is processed using non-incineration disinfection technology. This entails shredding and disinfecting the waste at specialised treatment plants. A small proportion of healthcare waste is technically hazardous and is sent abroad for incineration.

There are two categories of healthcare waste:

* **Non-risk waste –** More than 80 per cent of healthcare waste is non-risk waste, i.e. normal household and catering waste.
  > Waste materials include nappies, incontinence wear, stoma bags, clear oxygen tubing, urinary catheter tubing and bags, nasogastric tubing, non-contaminated gloves and aprons, etc. that are assessed as non-infectious.

* **Risk waste –** Ninety-five per cent of risk waste can be satisfactorily treated by non-incineration disinfection technology. Only 5 per cent requires incineration, e.g. body parts and blood, cytotoxic materials:
  > Potentially infectious waste, e.g. blood and items visibly soiled with blood
  > Contaminated waste from patients with transmissible infectious disease
  > Incontinence wear from patients with known or suspected infections
  > Items contaminated with body fluids other than faeces, urine or breast milk, e.g. pus, sputum or peritoneal fluid

> Anatomical waste, e.g. amputated body parts, placentas, removed growths such as benign cysts

> Sharps – injection needles, epidural and spinal needles, scalpels, etc.

> Radioactive waste – produced during the processing of X-rays

> Cytotoxic waste – produced during chemotherapy.

## SAFE DISPOSAL OF SHARPS

The term 'sharp' refers to any object which has been used in the diagnosis, treatment or prevention of disease that is likely to cause a puncture wound or cut to the skin, e.g. needles and syringes, intravenous cannula introducers, scalpels, stitch cutters, etc. (HSE, 2012). These items of waste are disposed of in a yellow rigid plastic container. This waste is shredded in a designated clinical waste disposal plant, treated with disinfectants and sent to landfill.

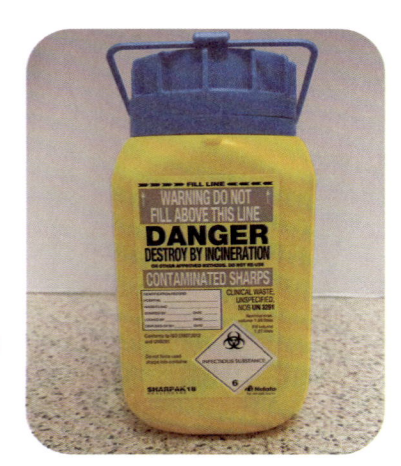

Some key points to remember are as follows:

* It is the responsibility of the person who uses a sharp to dispose of it safely.
* Syringes and needles should be disposed of as a single unit.
* Used sharps should be carefully discarded into designated sharps containers at the point of use.
* Sharps boxes should be securely stored out of the reach of clients, visitors and children.
* Needles should not be re-capped, bent, broken or disassembled.
* Sharps should never be passed from person to person.
* Sharps boxes should be closed when three-quarters full.

## NEEDLESTICK INJURIES

The healthcare environment is a dynamic one where unexpected events happen on a regular basis. Patients and staff can sometimes act unpredictably, often due to circumstances that may be beyond their control, and needlestick injuries can and do occur from time to time in healthcare. It is imperative that nurses know how to react when the unexpected happens. As in all aspects of healthcare delivery, safety is always the priority.

In the event of a nurse or other staff member or patient receiving a needlestick injury, the following procedure must be adhered to:

* Encourage the wound to bleed.
* Wash the wound with running water.
* Cover the wound with a waterproof dressing.
* Report the incident to the line manager.
* Follow local policy for documenting the incident.
* Post-exposure, the incident must be reported to the occupational health department, where advice in relation to testing and prophylactic treatment will be offered.

> **Remember!**
> - Bleed it!
> - Wash it!
> - Cover it!
> - Report it!
> - Never ignore it!

## SAFE MANAGEMENT OF ACCIDENTS AND SPILLAGES

Accidents and spillages can occur when caring for clients/patients and it is important to be prepared for this eventuality. The contents of a used commode or bedpan may spill or urine may spill during the routine emptying of a catheter bag. All blood and body fluid spillages should be dealt with immediately as they are high-risk incidents. Local policies and guidelines will dictate procedures; these are based on national guidelines.

## MANAGEMENT OF LINEN AND LAUNDRY

Linen or laundry that has been used in the healthcare environment can be categorised into the following three groups:

* Clean/unused linen
* Soiled linen
* Contaminated linen.

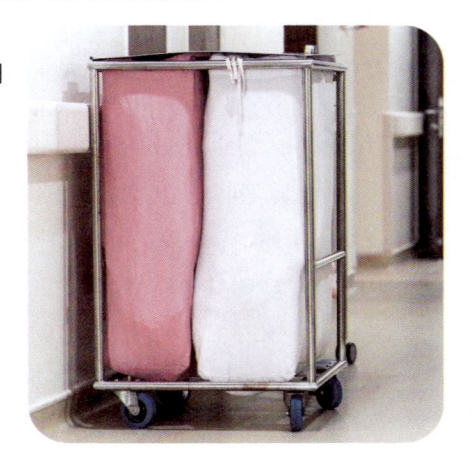

## CLEAN/UNUSED LINEN

This is linen that has been laundered and is ready for use. It must be stored in in a clean, closed cupboard, not in the sluice or bathroom. It must be segregated from soiled linen.

Clean linen should be delivered to wards or bedrooms in clean containers. If clean linen is taken into an isolation room and not used, it must be laundered again before use.

## SOILED LINEN

This is linen that is soiled in the normal way but not with potentially infectious bodily fluids or blood, e.g. normally soiled bed linen, bed linen with tea or porridge spills.

## CONTAMINATED LINEN

This is linen that has been contaminated with blood or potentially infectious bodily fluids, or bed linen that has been used by a patient with a known infection (soiled or not).

* Gloves and aprons should be worn when handling contaminated linen to avoid splashes on uniforms and contamination of hands.
* Gather infected linen so gross contamination is contained within the linen. This linen will be placed in a water-soluble bag – (an alginate bag).
* If two people are present, one holds the water-soluble bag open while the other places the contaminated linen inside.
* If only one person is present, hold the edge of the open end of the water-soluble bag in one hand and place soiled linen inside the bag with the other. Take care not to contaminate the outside of the bag.
* Tie the water-soluble bag using a tie or by knotting the edges.
* Place the water-soluble bag of contaminated linen into the designated (usually red) laundry bag.
* Remove PPE.
* Wash hands.

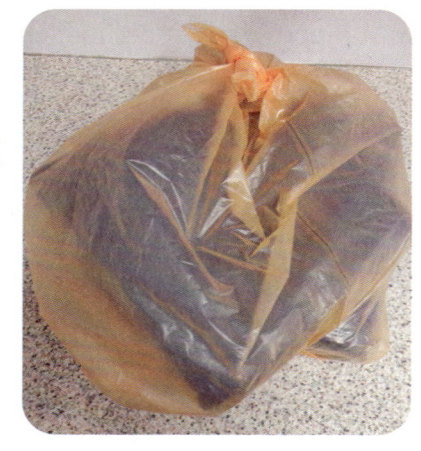

The water-soluble alginate bag will prevent contamination from soaking through the outer bag and this will protect the person handling the laundry bag. The alginate bag will be placed directly into the washing machine and will disintegrate in the hot water.

## PATIENT PLACEMENT

Traditionally, patients in hospitals have been cared for in wards where a number of patients are accommodated together, usually sharing bathroom facilities. With increased awareness in relation to infection prevention and control, more modern hospital facilities provide a larger proportion of single room accommodation with en-suite bathroom facilities. This is referred to as caring for a patient in isolation and it is recommended in both of the following situations:

* **Protective isolation –** for protecting a patient who is immunocompromised and at increased risk of contracting an infection by coming into contact with others.

* **Source isolation –** for protecting those either caring for or coming into contact with the patient. In this instance the patient is the source of the infection.

In both cases the patient will be allocated a single room with en-suite bathroom facilities. All nursing care will be provided within the confines of the room; the patient is not permitted to go outside the room unless to undergo investigations that require transportation to another area of the hospital.

The appropriate use of PPE will be required in both situations.

# REVISION QUESTIONS

1. Discuss the difference between the terms 'infection prevention' and 'infection control'.
2. Discuss, with your classmates, the importance of infection prevention and control practices in the healthcare setting for (a) patients, (b) staff and (c) visitors.
3. List the four main micro-organisms that cause infections.
4. Outline the ways in which micro-organisms can pass from person to person.
5. Describe the chain of infection, using coronavirus as an example.
6. What are standard precautions? List them.
7. Pick two standard precautions and describe how they are implemented in an acute hospital.
8. Differentiate between the three levels of decontamination.
9. List the two categories of waste generated in healthcare settings.

# 8

# Infectious Illnesses

In this chapter you will learn about:

* Blood-borne viruses
* Healthcare-associated infections (HCAIs)
* Transmission-based precautions

## Blood-borne viruses

Blood-borne viruses are carried in the blood. In some people they cause few or no symptoms, but in others they can cause severe illness and even death. Due to the nature of healthcare, workers are at risk of coming into contact with these viruses, so it is important that all categories of healthcare workers understand how to prevent cross-infection. Implementing standard precautions will prevent the spread of blood-borne viruses.

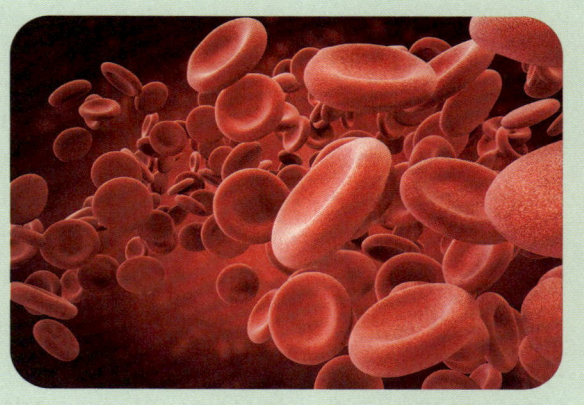

The most common blood-borne viruses are hepatitis B, hepatitis C and HIV (human immunodeficiency virus).

## HEPATITIS B

Hepatitis B is a virus that affects the liver and can cause serious illness. It can take six weeks to six months from the time of infection before symptoms appear. It can cause fever, nausea, tiredness, a swollen abdomen and jaundice. There is no specific treatment other than rest, good nutrition and avoidance of alcohol.

Some people who get hepatitis B continue to carry the virus in their blood even though they appear well. This is called chronic hepatitis B and the people who have it are referred to as carriers. They may feel healthy and not show any evidence of liver damage. Some people develop more severe liver disease, such as liver scarring (cirrhosis), liver failure or cancer. Some carriers do not know they have hepatitis B and they may spread the virus to others without knowing

In the healthcare setting, hepatitis B is prevented from spreading from patients to healthcare workers by vaccinating healthcare workers and implementing standard precautions. Since 2008 Hepatitis B vaccine is given to all babies as part of the 6-in-1 vaccine that is given at two, four and six months of age.

Hepatitis B is much more infectious than other blood-borne viruses.

## HEPATITIS C

Hepatitis C is a viral infection that causes inflammation of the liver. About 25 per cent of people who are infected clear the virus within one year of infection. The remaining 75 per cent develop chronic (long-term) infection. This can cause serious liver disease, including cirrhosis (scarring of the liver) and liver cancer. This liver damage occurs gradually over 20–30 years in people with chronic infection.

There is no vaccine to protect against hepatitis C, but new treatments have become available in recent years and over 90 per cent of people who are infected can be cured. In the healthcare setting prevention of the spread of hepatitis C is achieved by implementing standard precautions.

## HIV AND AIDS

HIV is the virus that causes AIDS (acquired immune deficiency syndrome). HIV attacks certain white blood cells called CD4 cells. When the CD4 count is low, the body's immune system is very weak and cannot fight off infections and diseases caused by viruses and bacteria.

A person with HIV may have no symptoms and may appear completely healthy for a long period of time. The only way to determine for sure whether infection is present is to be tested for HIV. The HIV antibody test looks for the presence of antibodies (disease-fighting proteins) to the virus in a person's blood. Someone with HIV antibodies is infected with the virus.

There is currently no vaccine to protect against becoming infected with HIV; however, the prognosis for infected people has improved greatly due to the development of highly active anti-retroviral therapy.

AIDS is the advanced stage of HIV infection. A person first becomes HIV infected and later, in most cases, develops AIDS. HIV can weaken the immune system to the point where the person has difficulty fighting off certain diseases, many of which are not normally a threat to a healthy person. A person receives an AIDS diagnosis from a doctor after developing one or more specific opportunistic infections, also known as AIDS indicator illnesses, which include severe pneumonia, several forms of cancer, damage to the brain and nervous system, and extreme weight loss.

# Healthcare-associated infections

A healthcare-associated infection (HCAI) is an infection that is acquired after contact with the healthcare services. This occurs most frequently after treatment in a hospital, but it can also happen after treatment in outpatient clinics, nursing homes and other healthcare settings. As a result of the rapid turnover of patients in acute healthcare settings, complex care is increasingly being delivered in the community.

The five most common HCAIs are:

* surgical site infection
* pneumonia
* urinary tract infection
* bloodstream infection
* gastroenteritis.

Healthcare associated infections can occur anywhere that a pathogen has an opportunity to invade the body. Some common sites are the urinary tract via the urethra, the respiratory tract, surgical wound sites and sites where invasive devices are in situ, e.g. intravenous catheters. Pathogens that invade the digestive system can cause vomiting and diarrhoea.

## CONSEQUENCES OF HCAIS

The consequences of contracting an HCAI can range from mild to moderate. If the infection has been caused by resistant bacteria it can be difficult to treat and a mild illness may progress to a moderate or severe illness. The symptoms of the disease will depend on the type of micro-organism causing the disease and the area of the body that has been invaded.

The infection may prolong the hospital stay and may involve the client taking medicines that would not otherwise be necessary. Prolonged stays in hospital will have financial implications for the individual and for the healthcare system itself. Contracting an HCAI can affect the person psychologically. It may cause stress and anxiety. The person may be concerned that they will not recover or that the infection will lead to death. The financial costs associated with the infection may also cause stress. In some cases, the individual and their family may experience stigma associated with having an infection that has the potential to spread to others, whether other users of the health services or family or friends.

Four of the most common HCAIs in Ireland are *Clostridioides difficile*, *Staphylococcus aureus*, MRSA and norovirus.

## CLOSTRIDIOIDES DIFFICILE

*Clostridioides difficile* (*C.diff*, formerly known as *Clostridium difficile*) is a bacterium that normally lives in the large intestine. A small proportion (less than 1 in 20) of the healthy adult population carry a small amount of *Clostridioides difficile* in their large intestine and do not experience any problem with it. It is kept in check by the normal, 'good' bacteria of the intestine.

However, when an antibiotic is taken, particularly a broad-spectrum antibiotic, some of the 'good' bacteria are also destroyed by the antibiotic, giving the bacteria an opportunity to multiply; subsequently an infection in the large intestine can occur. Most cases of *C. diff* are associated with previous antibiotic use (Baxter *et al.* 2008).

The symptoms of *C. diff* infection are: diarrhoea with a very distinctive, offensive odour; loss of appetite, nausea and stomach cramps. Fever can occur. Most people only get mildly ill and recover fully, but in certain circumstances the person may get seriously ill and develop colitis (inflammation of the bowel). If the colitis is severe it can be life-threatening.

People most at risk of developing *Clostridioides difficile* infection are:

- those taking antibiotics, particularly long term
- those who are immunosuppressed
- the elderly
- someone who has recently undergone bowel surgery
- those with a chronic underlying condition.

Infection is spread by the faecal–oral route. Diagnosis is by testing a specimen of faeces. Treatment may be cessation of the current antibiotic therapy and commencement of antibiotic therapy specific to the *C. diff* bacterium.

## STAPHYLOCOCCUS AUREUS

*Staphylococcus aureus* is a common pathogenic bacterium that can cause a wide variety of infections, both in hospital and in community settings. It is commonly carried on the skin and in the nose, where it mostly causes no harm (colonisation). It has been documented that 30 per cent of people continuously carry *S. aureus* in their noses, while many other people carry the bacteria, without any ill effects, from time to time (HPSC, 2018).

*S. aureus* is mainly spread by direct person-to-person contact (e.g. on unwashed hands) or through indirect contact by touching objects that have been contaminated with the bacteria. It is only rarely transmitted through the air. Infections can be localised (confined to one part of the body) or generalised (spread to many parts of the body). Most are relatively minor and do not cause a person to become very ill (for example, a boil or an infected cut in the skin). In rare cases it can cause more severe infections that may require treatment in hospital.

Infections caused by *S. aureus* include as follows:

- Infected skin wounds or cuts
- Boils
- Impetigo
- Cellulitis (a type of skin infection)
- Urinary tract infection ('cystitis')
- Sinus infections
- Pneumonia
- Bone and joint infections.

Most strains of *S. aureus* are treated with penicillin-type antibiotics.

## METHICILLIN-RESISTANT *STAPHYLOCOCCUS AUREUS*

Methicillin-resistant *Staphylococcus aureus* (MRSA) is a subgroup of *Staphylococcus aureus* that is resistant to a range of antibiotics, including penicillin antibiotics. MRSA first appeared in 1961, soon after the introduction of the antibiotic methicillin (which is no longer in use). Since then, MRSA has spread widely in many countries and has been particularly associated with hospitals and other healthcare facilities.

MRSA is resistant to most types of antibiotics, but most MRSA strains can be treated with antibiotics such as vancomycin and teicoplanin, and these are usually the drugs of choice for treating serious MRSA infections.

In general, MRSA infections tend to occur in older hospital patients and those with the most severe underlying illnesses. The following are considered to be important risk factors for invasive MRSA infection:

* Age (older age groups are more prone)
* Gender (males are twice as at risk as females)
* Prolonged hospital stay
* Patients in intensive care, surgical and burns units
* Patients with diabetes and other chronic conditions
* Patients treated with broad-spectrum antibiotics.

The MRSA bacteria will have been identified from a swab or other specimen taken typically from the nose, groin or any surgical wound site.

Patients with MRSA are usually moved to a single room or dedicated isolation ward to prevent the spread of the organism to other patients and staff.

Staff will wear gloves and gowns to help prevent contamination of their skin and clothes (and thus further spread of the bacteria to other patients and staff members). Gloves and gowns should be changed for each patient encounter.

Good hygiene is essential for the control of MRSA and other infections. Staff and visitors alike should be careful to wash their hands thoroughly before and after visiting a patient.

## NOROVIRUS

Norovirus is one of the most common causes of gastroenteritis. Outbreaks in busy places such as hospitals, nursing homes and schools are common because the virus can survive for several days on surfaces or objects touched by an infected person. Norovirus is also commonly known as the winter vomiting bug.

Symptoms include:

- nausea (often sudden onset)
- vomiting (often projectile)
- watery diarrhoea.

Norovirus is very contagious and can spread easily from person to person. Both the faeces and vomit of an infected person contain the virus and are infectious. People infected with norovirus are contagious from the moment they begin feeling ill to two or three days after recovery. Some people may be contagious for as long as two weeks after recovery.

The faecal–oral route of transmission is the most common. This may include contact with contaminated surfaces or objects and then touching the mouth or mucous membranes. Consuming contaminated food or water can also lead to the spread and occurrence of norovirus.

In hospitals, healthcare workers and hospital visitors can spread the virus to other patients or contaminate surfaces through hand contact.

In recent years, a significant number of hospitals and nursing homes in Ireland have reported outbreaks of the winter vomiting bug, which has caused stress not only to sufferers and staff but also to other patients and residents. During an outbreak it is necessary to restrict visiting and the movement of people into and out of the healthcare facility.

## VANCOMYCIN-RESISTANT ENTEROCOCCI

Vancomycin-resistant enterococci (VRE) are bacteria that live in the bowel and that are resistant to certain antibiotics, e.g. vancomycin. For most people VRE live harmlessly in the bowel and do not cause infection. However, when people become immunosuppressed VRE can multiply and cause infections such as kidney infections, wound infections and, in severe cases, sepsis. VRE infection is difficult to treat because of its resistance to antibiotics.

VRE spreads through direct or indirect contact. People who have undergone prolonged antibiotic treatment are at increased risk of becoming infected. In 2014, Ireland had the highest proportion of VRE bloodstream infection in Europe (HSE/HPSC, 2015).

## CPE AND CRE

In Ireland, the terms carbapenemase-producing *Enterobacteriaceae* (CPE) and carbapenem-resistant *Enterobacteriaceae* (CRE) are often used interchangeably by healthcare workers when referring to a family of bacteria that live in the bowel. CPE/CRE have developed the ability to become resistant to last-resort powerful antimicrobials known as carbapenems, which makes them more challenging to treat if they go on to cause infection. CRE is another strand of bacteria that has developed resistance to antibiotics. The effects and the mode of transmission is similar to VRE.

# Transmission-based precautions

Transmission-based precautions are additional measures that are required when standard precautions may not be sufficient to prevent the transmission of certain infectious agents. While standard precautions apply to all patients, transmission-based precautions apply to particular patients who have either a suspected or a confirmed infectious illness.

These additional precautions include measures to prevent airborne, droplet and contact transmission of infectious agents (HSE 2009).

Transmission-based precautions are used **in addition to** standard precautions and they should be applied in the following circumstances:

* When a patient has an active infection
* Where a patient is not yet experiencing any symptoms but is suspected to be infectious or incubating an infection
* When a patient is known to be colonised with a pathogenic micro-organism.

Risk assessment is important to identify patients who require transmission-based precautions. Risk assessment is carried out at ward level and at management level. Communication between staff is a fundamental part of risk assessment. All signs and symptoms of infection should be noted and reported. Remember, good observation skills are a fundamental aspect of the provision of effective healthcare. The decision to implement transmission-based precautions is taken by the infection prevention and control team.

Some infections are spread by more than one route and will require a combination of precautions, e.g. for influenza, both contact and droplet precautions are required.

## CONTACT PRECAUTIONS

These precautions are applied, in addition to standard precautions, to prevent the transmission of highly transmissible organisms that are transmitted through both direct contact and indirect contact.

Contact controls are as follows:

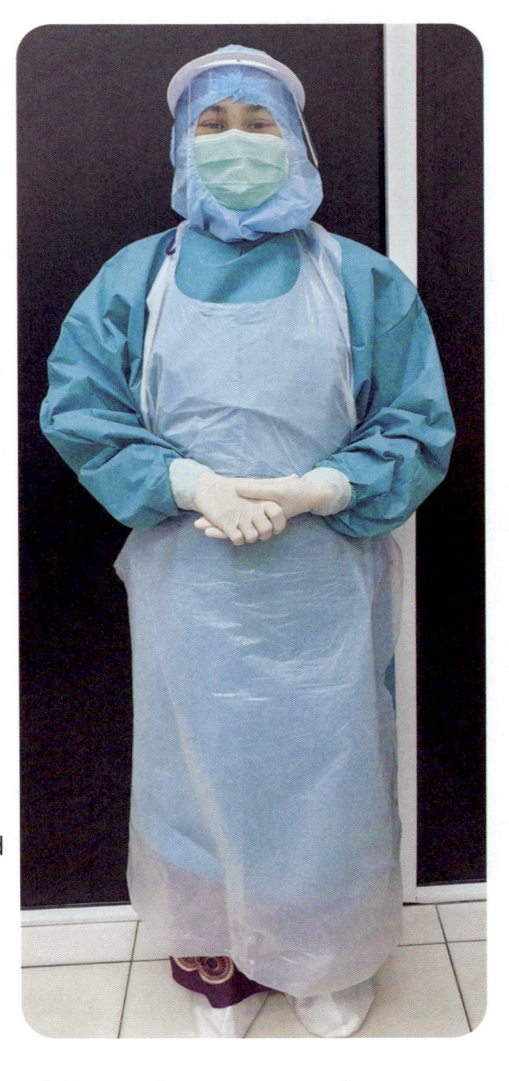

* The patient should be cared for in a single room with en-suite bathroom facilities.

* Stringent adherence to handwashing guidelines – soap and water is preferable to alcohol gel.

* PPE – gown and gloves should be worn by healthcare personnel for all interactions. This protective equipment should be put on before entering the room and should be taken off and disposed of before leaving the room.

* Care of patient/client equipment – the patient should have their own dedicated equipment, e.g. thermometer, blood pressure monitor, etc. Single-use disposable equipment should be used where possible. Essential items only should be in the room.

* Avoid taking charts into the room. These should be stored safely outside the room, perhaps on a trolley outside the door, and should be filled in when PPE has been removed. Remember to ensure that patient confidentiality is protected at all times.

* Decontamination of equipment and the environment – daily cleaning with water and detergent should be carried out, as well as disinfection with a chlorine-based solution (1,000 ppm).

* At discharge, terminal cleaning of the room should be carried out.

## AIRBORNE PRECAUTIONS

These precautions are applied, in addition to standard precautions, to prevent the transmission of infectious organisms that are transmitted via the air from one person to another.

Airborne precautions prevent transmission of pathogens of small particle size that remain infectious over long distances when suspended in the air.

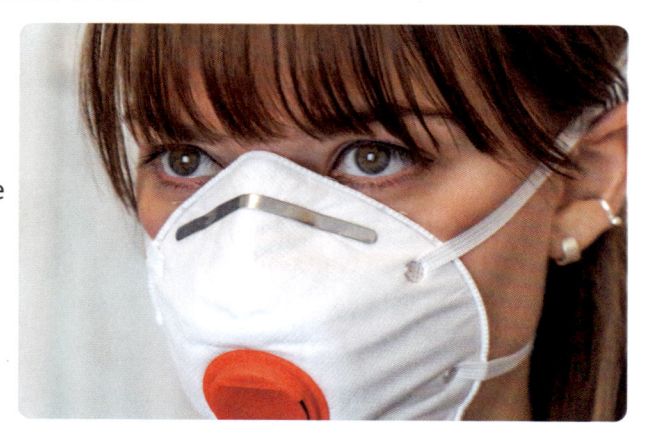

Airborne controls are as follows:

* The patient should be cared for in a single room with adequate air exchanges per hour.

* PPE – staff should use appropriate face masks to prevent the tiny particles being breathed in. Masks with a protection rating of FFP2 or FFP3 will offer greater protection than a regular paper surgical mask. These must be correctly fitted prior to entering the room and removed after leaving the room. Gloves and apron should be worn during direct contact with resident.

* Patient movement should be restricted. As far as possible, any examinations or tests, e.g. chest X-rays, should be carried out in the room. If the patient needs to leave the room they should wear a surgical face mask to help prevent respiratory secretions being discharged.

* Care of patient/client equipment – the patient should have their own dedicated equipment, e.g. thermometer, blood pressure monitor, etc. Single-use disposable equipment should be used where possible. Essential items only should be in the room.

* Avoid taking charts into the room. These should be stored safely outside the room, perhaps on a trolley outside the door, and should be filled in when PPE has been removed. Remember to ensure that patient confidentiality is protected at all times.

- Decontamination of equipment and the environment – daily cleaning with water and detergent should be carried out, as well as disinfection with a chlorine-based solution (1,000 ppm).
- At discharge, terminal cleaning of the room should be carried out.

## DROPLET PRECAUTIONS

These precautions are applied, in addition to standard precautions, to prevent the transmission of infective organisms that are transmitted via large droplets of respiratory secretions from one person directly onto a mucosal surface of another (e.g. eyes, nose, mouth). Droplets are shed through coughing, sneezing, talking and during procedures like respiratory suctioning.

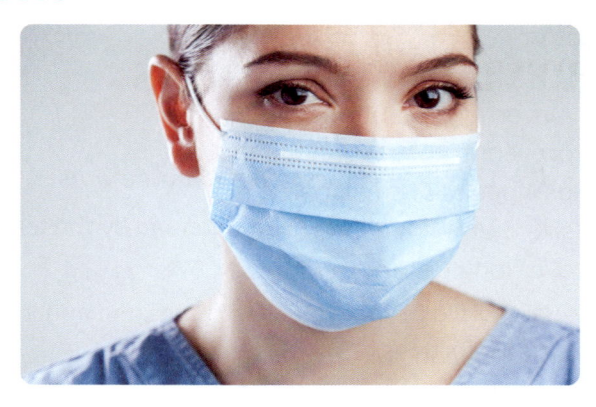

Droplet controls are as follows:

- The patient should be cared for in a single room. If a single room is not available, infected patients should be cohorted, away from non-infected patients.
- Alternatively, spatial separation of more than three feet is required and drawing the curtain between client beds is very important.
- PPE – surgical masks should be worn if within three feet of the patient. Gloves and apron should be worn when in direct contact with the patient.
- If the patient needs to leave the room they should wear a surgical face mask to help prevent respiratory secretions being discharged. Limit movement to essential purposes only.
- Care of patient/client equipment – the patient should have their own dedicated equipment, e.g. thermometer, blood pressure monitor, etc. Single-use disposable equipment should be used where possible. Essential items only should be in the room.
- Avoid taking charts into the room. These should be stored safely outside the room, perhaps on a trolley outside the door, and should be filled in

when PPE has been removed. Remember to ensure that patient confidentiality is protected at all times.

* Decontamination of equipment and the environment – daily cleaning with water and detergent should be carried out, as well as disinfection with a chlorine-based solution (1,000 ppm).

* At discharge, terminal cleaning of the room should be carried out.

## REVISION QUESTIONS

1. List three common blood-borne viruses.
2. Describe what you understand by the term 'healthcare-associated infection'.
3. Discuss, with your classmates, the implications of healthcare-associated infections.
4. What are transmission-based precautions?
5. Select a common infection and describe the relevant transmission-based precautions associated with it.

# Fluid Balance

In this chapter you will learn about:

* Normal fluid balance
* Dehydration
* Fluid overload
* Fluid balance
* Measuring and recording fluid balance using a fluid balance chart

## Normal fluid balance

The human body is made up of 60–70% water. Water is vital for good health, it is necessary to control body temperature, for the delivery of nutrients and gases to cells, and for removing waste products from the body. Fluid is taken into the body by drinking and in food. Water is excreted from the body in urine, faeces and through sweat and expired air.

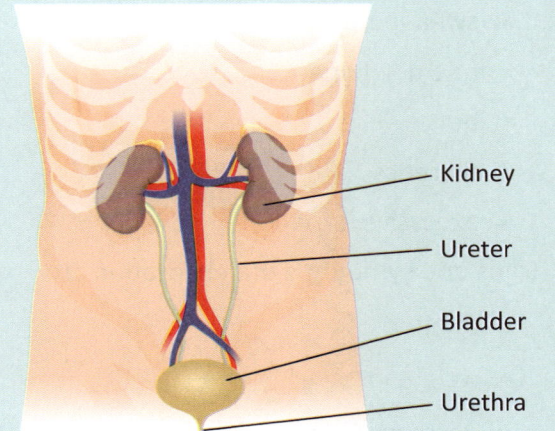

— Kidney

— Ureter

— Bladder

— Urethra

The balance between fluid intake and output is regulated by the kidneys. The body has a natural inclination to achieve homeostasis or balance in all its systems. Where homeostasis is maintained, the intake of fluid equals the fluid excreted by the body, thereby maintaining optimal hydration.

A fluid intake of 1.5–2 litres in twenty-four hours is recommended for adults (roughly six to eight glasses of water daily). The **minimum** amount of urine produced that is necessary to remove essential waste products from the body is 500 ml in twenty-four hours (Grant & Waugh 2018).

Average urine output is 1.5 litres plus

- 100 ml in faeces
- 400 ml from sweating
- 400 ml from the lungs

in twenty-four hours.

If fluid intake is insufficient or if fluid output is excessive, dehydration can occur.

# Dehydration

Dehydration occurs when the fluid output exceeds the fluid intake. This is referred to as having a negative fluid balance.

Dehydration can be caused by:

- diarrhoea
- vomiting
- sweating/fever
- haemorrhage
- burns
- diuretics
- excessive urination.

Signs and symptoms of dehydration are:

- thirst
- weight loss
- decreased urinary output
- dry skin and mucous membranes
- fatigue.

Clinically, dehydration can cause an increase in body temperature, an increase in pulse rate and a drop in blood pressure (Dougherty *et al.* 2015).

Dehydration is common among older people and is often not recognised or considered significant, yet it impairs cognitive function, causes headaches, tiredness and dizziness, and reduces alertness. Older people, particularly those with dementia or those who have suffered a stroke may have a reduced thirst sensitivity and this can increase the likelihood of them becoming dehydrated.

Illness can affect the fluid balance of the body. Someone who is breathless will lose more fluid through breathing. Someone with a high temperature will lose more fluid through sweating. Vomiting and diarrhoea can cause rapid fluid loss.

### EMPATHIC BEHAVIOUR

Listening to people and observing them will help the nurse to recognise signs of dehydration.

* A person might be asking for their water jug to be refilled frequently or for assistance to go to the bathroom more often than is usual for them.
* The nurse might observe that the person has sunken eyes, that their skin is dry or that their mouth is very dry when they are chatting.
* The nurse might notice that the person is more tired than usual or that they are disorientated or confused.

# Fluid overload

Fluid overload is a positive fluid balance when the circulating fluid volume is excessive. It can be caused by:

* congestive cardiac failure
* renal failure
* high sodium intake
* cirrhosis of the liver
* excessive infusion of intravenous fluids

Signs and symptoms of fluid overload are:

* an increase in the person's weight
* swelling and oedema in different parts of the body, e.g. puffiness around the eyes or in the ankles or lower back
* breathlessness.

> **EMPATHIC BEHAVIOUR**
>
> Listening to people and observing them will help the nurse to recognise signs of fluid overload.
>
> A person might, when asked, say that they are not thirsty. The nurse might observe areas of puffiness or swelling.

# Measuring fluid balance

In nursing practice, this refers to the procedure of measuring fluid intake and output to determine fluid balance. This information can be recorded on a fluid balance chart.

As with any procedure, it is essential to explain to the person that you are monitoring their fluid intake and output. A full and clear explanation will assist in compliance and so maximise accuracy.

The person will need to inform the nurse of the amount of fluid taken and the time it was taken at. Good-quality therapeutic relationships are the foundation for success in procedures where the person and the nurse work together to accurately gather essential data.

When assessing fluid intake, the aim is to gain information on the amount, time and type of fluid consumed. If the person is taking fluids via a feeding tube or intravenously the nurse will include these on the fluid balance chart.

The person will need to pass urine into a commode so that it can be measured by the nurse. If the person has a urinary catheter, the nurse will empty it into a measuring jug and the amount will be entered on the fluid balance chart.

All outputs will be measured and recorded, e.g. fluid lost in surgical drains, fluid draining from nasogastric tubes, fluid lost during bowel motions, etc.

Fluid intake and output are calculated over a twenty-four-hour period. This usually commences at 8 a.m. (0800 hours: observations are always documented using the twenty-four-hour clock).

# MEASURING AND RECORDING FLUID INTAKE AND OUTPUT USING A FLUID BALANCE CHART

The following are examples of when it is necessary to monitor fluid balance:

* Any patient who has undergone surgery
* Any patient who is acutely ill
* Any patient who has shown signs or symptoms of fluid imbalance.

## Exercise

Discuss in groups the different causes of fluid imbalance, both overhydration and dehydration.

The decision to monitor fluid balance will be a multidisciplinary one, including, for example, the nurse, the doctor and the dietitian. It is the responsibility of the nurse to ensure that the procedure is done accurately. Before beginning fluid monitoring it is important that the person is educated about the fact that monitoring is being carried out and that a fluid balance chart is being used to do this. Understanding and co-operation is vital for the accurate monitoring of fluid balance.

## EMPATHIC BEHAVIOUR

When providing information and education to people it is important to explain things in a way that is understanable to the person. A good-quality therapeutic relationship between the nurse and the person will facilitate this.

* Using vocabulary that the person is familiar with will be much more effective than using medical jargon that they may not understand.
* Allowing the person opportunities to ask questions is important and will make them feel more in control of their situation.
* Safeguarding privacy and dignity is especially important when measuring urine and bodily fluids.
* The nurse needs to be aware of the sensitivities of the person and a partnership approach to care must be taken at all times.
* The nurse and the person have shared goals: to accurately measure and record the person's input and output.

## RECORDING FLUID INTAKE

When commencing a fluid balance chart it is important to accurately record the person's name and other uniquely identifying pieces of information on the chart. It will also be necessary to accurately record the date.

* Fluid intake must include all fluids that the patient takes into the body. This includes all liquids, any ice, liquid foods such as soup and ice cream, any intravenous infusions and any fluids administered through feeding tubes.
* Measure all fluids taken in.
* Record, in the appropriate place in the chart, the time and amount of fluids taken.
* Record intake over a twenty-four-hour period using the twenty-four-hour clock when recording.
* Add together all fluid intake over the twenty-four-hour period.

## RECORDING FLUID OUTPUT

Fluid output must include all fluids that the patient passes out of the body. This includes all liquids, e.g. urine, vomit, diarrhoea and any volumes from drains following surgery.

* Measure all fluid output.
* Record, in the appropriate place in the chart, the time and volume of fluids put out.
* Record output over a twenty-four-hour period – use the twenty-four-hour clock.
* Add together all fluid output over the twenty-four-hour period.

## CALCULATING THE BALANCE

* Total intake in twenty-four hours is balanced against total output in twenty-four hours.
* When intake is greater than output there will be a positive balance.
* When output is greater than intake there will be a negative balance.
* The calculated balance will always be recorded and reported to the supervising nurse.

(See Appendix 2 Fluid Balance Chart)

# Fluid balance practice

## PRACTICE CASE STUDY 1

Ann is a resident in Sunflower Nursing Home. She has recently been found to have a kidney infection. This frequently results in an increased urge to urinate, which has led to Ann becoming incontinent. Ann now has a urinary catheter. It is important to monitor Ann's intake and output in this situation. It is wise to encourage her to drink as much fluid as possible to help flush her kidneys, and it is important to measure her output to ensure that her kidney function is adequate.

*Fill out a fluid balance chart in relation to Ann's situation:*

- Morning: catheter emptied 650 ml urine
- Breakfast: 100 ml milk + rice krispies
- Mid-morning: 250 ml tea
- Noon: 175 ml MiWadi + lunch
- Mid-afternoon: 300 ml tea and 7UP
- Mid-afternoon: catheter emptied, 210 ml drained
- Supper: 120 ml tea
- Evening: 220 ml 7 Up
- Night: catheter emptied, 175 ml drained

*Identify whether Ann has a positive or negative fluid balance for this twenty-four-hour period.*

## PRACTICE CASE STUDY 2

Shane is a twenty-five-year-old man who is suffering from vomiting. His hydration levels are a concern, so it is important to monitor his fluid balance. He has been asked to urinate in disposable urinals, which are collected by the nurse and measured prior to disposal. Because of his persistent vomiting he has intravenous fluids infusing at 80 ml/hr.

*Fill out a fluid balance chart in relation to Shane's situation:*

- IV fluids: 80 ml/hr … continuous infusion for twelve hours
- Morning: vomited 80 ml clear fluid
- Morning: drank 35 ml water
- Noon: urinated 340 ml
- Noon: drank 70 ml 7 Up
- Noon: vomited 55 ml clear fluid
- 3 p.m.: drank 25 ml water
- 4 p.m.: vomited 120 ml
- 6 p.m.: urinated 190 ml
- 8 p.m.: drank 125 ml 7 Up

*Identify whether Shane has a positive or negative fluid balance for this twenty-four-hour period.*

## PRACTICE CASE STUDY 3

Pat Ryan is eighty-four years of age and has been admitted to the medical ward in a confused state. He has a history of diarrhoea and vomiting and although the symptoms have subsided his confusion may be due to his dehydrated state.

He was admitted early in the morning and immediately an intravenous cannula was inserted, and he was given 90 ml of normal saline per hour from 8 a.m. until 4 p.m. (eight hours).

At 12 midday he passed 300 ml of urine into a urinal and by this time his mental state was much improved. At 1 p.m. he had his dinner and a glass of water (180 ml). After dinner he had a nap and when he woke up at 3 p.m. he asked for a bowl of jelly and ice cream (200 ml). At 4 p.m. he went to the toilet again and passed 300 ml of urine.

At teatime Pat had some sausages and rashers and drank two cups of tea with his meal (150 ml each). At 7 p.m. he went to the toilet and passed 400 ml of urine. While he was in the bathroom, he felt unwell again and he vomited 100 ml into a bowl. At 10 p.m. the nurse brought him his night medications and he took them with half a glass of water (75 ml). Pat fell asleep at midnight.

Pat is an early riser and he woke up at 6 a.m. and went to the toilet, where he passed 250 ml of urine. When the nurse came around with his tablets at 6 a.m. he took them with half a glass of water (75 ml). Pat was feeling much better when he woke up. He loves to start the day with a cup of tea so the health care assistant made him one before breakfast came around (150 ml).

*Fill out a fluid balance chart for Pat, calculating whether he has a positive or negative fluid balance at the end of the twenty-four-hour period.*

## PRACTICE CASE STUDY 4

Brigid has been a resident in Sunflower Nursing Home for six months. She usually enjoys the food and drinks in the home, and she particularly likes the constant supply of fresh iced water that is available in the sitting room. Unfortunately for Brigid, she recently contracted the winter vomiting bug.

At 8 a.m. Brigid had her breakfast and drank a cup of tea. At mid-morning she had a small glass of water. She went to the bathroom at 11 a.m. and passed 200 ml of urine.

At dinner time Brigid had a bowl of soup and another small glass of water with her meal. After dinner she took a nap.

Brigid woke at 2 p.m. and went to the bathroom, where she passed 200 ml of urine. The health care assistant offered her a cup of tea and a biscuit at 3 p.m., which she enjoyed. At around 5 p.m. Brigid started to feel unwell. She ate a small chicken sandwich at teatime but did not feel like drinking anything. Shortly afterwards she complained of cramps in her tummy.

At 7 p.m. she asked the health care assistant to walk her to the bathroom as she felt very unwell. While in the bathroom she had a bout of diarrhoea (200 ml).

The health care assistant helped her back into bed and left a bowl beside her as Brigid felt quite sick. At 9 p.m. she vomited 150 ml into the bowl. The health care assistant was concerned about Brigid as she was unable to take anything orally due to her illness, so she reported the changes in Brigid's condition to the staff nurse, who came to review her.

While the nurse was there Brigid had another bout of vomiting (200 ml). Both the HCA and the nurse were concerned that Brigid would become dehydrated as she was taking very little orally and because of her episodes of vomiting and diarrhoea. They decided to call the doctor, who came and prescribed 100 ml of saline hourly for Brigid. The nurse inserted the intravenous catheter at 11 p.m. and started the infusion.

At midnight Brigid had another episode of diarrhoea and passed 250 ml. She fell asleep after that and woke at 5 a.m. feeling somewhat better. At 6 a.m. she passed 200 ml of urine into the commode.

At 7 a.m. she felt much better and had a small glass of water. The HCA reported the improvement in Brigid's condition to the nurse and they decided they would call the doctor to see if they could discontinue the intravenous infusion.

**Fill out a fluid balance chart for Brigid, calculating whether she has a positive or negative balance at the end of the twenty-four-hour period.**

# Physiological Observations

**10**

In this chapter you will learn about:

* Measuring and recording body temperature
* Measuring and recording pulse
* Measuring and recording respiration
* Pulse oximetry
* Measuring and recording blood pressure
* Early warning system (EWS)
* Recording physiological observations on the INEWS chart

## Observations/Vital signs

### DEFINITION

**Observation** refers to the physiological observations that are measured during the assessment of a person. Sometimes these are referred to as **vital signs**. This refers specifically to the physical measuring of temperature, pulse, respiration, pulse oximetry and blood pressure.

Taking patient observations is a fundamental nursing skill. The interpretation of the measurements taken is vital in determining the level of care provided, whether a treatment or intervention is necessary and preventing a patient deteriorating.

Manual and sometimes highly technical equipment can be used to measure vital signs; however, it is important for nurses to use their senses in observing changes in a patient's condition.

> ### Exercise
>
> * Considering the senses of sight and smell, what might a nurse observe about a patient that would indicate that they had a high temperature?
> * Considering the senses of sight and hearing, what might a nurse observe about a patient that would indicate that they were having difficulty breathing?
> * Considering the senses of sight and touch, what might a nurse observe about a patient that would indicate that they had a low temperature?

# Measuring and recording body temperature

> ### DEFINITION
>
> **Body temperature** represents the balance between heat production and heat loss. All body tissues produce heat, depending on how metabolically active they are. Body temperature is regulated by the hypothalamus in the brain. Humans have the ability, through homeostasis, to maintain a constant body temperature despite environmental changes. The body core generally has the highest temperature while the skin has the coolest.

**Normal body temperature** falls into the range of 36.1–38°C, but this may vary, by as much as 0.6°C, according to the site used for measurement. Core body temperature can be more than 0.4°C higher than oral temperature and more than 0.2°C lower than rectal temperature. A temperature above 41°C can cause convulsions and the body cannot sustain a temperature above 43°C (Dougherty *et al.* 2015).

**Hypothermia** occurs when body temperature falls below 35°C. This fall in temperature causes the metabolic rate to decrease. As the temperature decreases, so too does the body's need for oxygen. This can lead to a reduction in respiratory rate.

Hypothermia can arise as a result of:

* environmental exposure
* medications that alter the perception of cold, or inhibit heat generation, or cause heat loss through vasodilation
* netabolic conditions, e.g. hypoglycaemia
* the exposure of internal organs during major surgery.

**Hyperthermia/pyrexia** is the name given to a rise in body temperature above 38°C. An elevation in temperature often indicates that infection is present.

## WHY DO WE MEASURE BODY TEMPERATURE?

Measuring body temperature is a fundamental skill in nursing practice. It is measured for the following reasons:

* To establish a baseline temperature, e.g. when a patient is admitted to hospital. This allows the nurse to make comparisons in subsequent measurements and so monitor changes in the person's condition.
* Post-operative fluctuations in temperature may indicate developing infection or the presence of a deep venous thrombosis.
* People who are immunosuppressed are less able to respond to infection and an invading bacterium could result in the development of sepsis.
* To monitor signs of incompatibility when a person is receiving a blood transfusion.
* To monitor the temperature of a person being treated for an infection – it is an indicator of the response to the treatment.
* To monitor the temperature of people recovering from hypothermia.

The frequency of measuring and recording will depend on the reason for monitoring and on the person's condition.

# EQUIPMENT

## DISPOSABLE THERMOMETERS

There are a variety of disposable thermometers available. The two most common are the chemical dot thermometer and the liquid crystal heat-sensitive strip. They are for single use only. The manufacturer's instructions must be followed to ensure an accurate reading. These thermometers tend to be used mostly in a domestic setting.

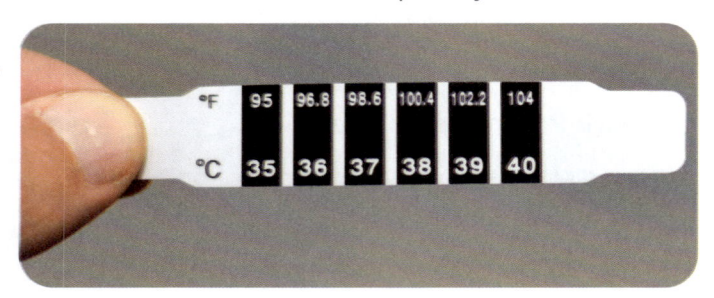

## DIGITAL THERMOMETERS

These can be used for measuring temperature using the oral cavity or the axilla. The probe is inserted into either of these areas and the reading is displayed digitally on the display screen.

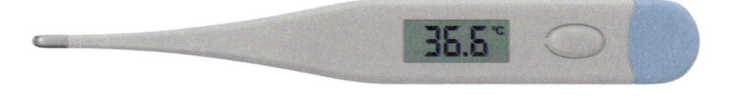

Cleaning the probe with an alcohol solution is necessary after each usage to prevent cross-infection.

## TYMPANIC THERMOMETERS

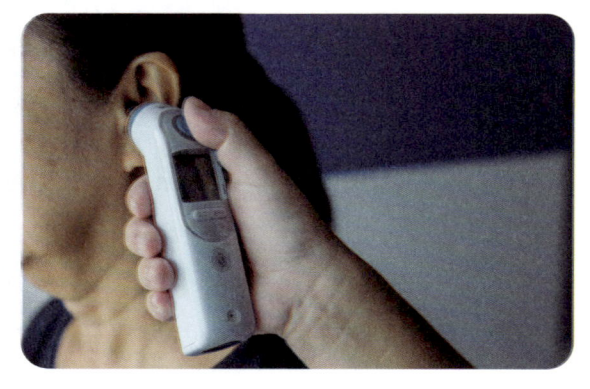

Tympanic thermometers have a probe with a disposable cover that is inserted into the external auditory canal. They detect infrared energy that is emitted from the tympanic membrane and surrounding tissue, which is displayed digitally as a temperature reading. The tympanic temperature correlates well with the core temperature, which is thought to be because the tympanic membrane shares its blood supply with the hypothalamus.

The thermometer must be covered by a disposable cover in order to function, and the detection window must be kept clean in order to obtain an accurate result. False readings may arise from incorrect technique, a damaged lens or inaccurate timing between measurements.

## METHODS OF MEASUREMENT

Traditionally, the mouth, axilla, rectum and external auditory canal have been the preferred sites for obtaining temperature readings, due to their accessibility. As temperature readings between these sites can vary it is important to use the same site continuously to allow for accurate comparisons.

### ORAL CAVITY

* Wash hands.
* Help the person into a comfortable position so that they will be able to tolerate the temperature probe.
* Place the clean thermometer under the person's tongue so that the probe lies adjacent to the frenulum at the junction of the floor of the mouth and the base of the tongue, on either the right or left side.
* Explain the importance of closing only the lips around the thermometer (not biting it), so that the oral temperature is maintained and not distorted by the inspiration of air through the mouth.
* Leave the thermometer in position for the required time.
* Read the temperature measured by the thermometer.
* Ensure that the person is left feeling as comfortable as possible to reassure them and reduce anxiety.
* Clean or dispose of equipment as appropriate.
* Wash hands.
* Accurately document the temperature reading.

## AXILLA

- Wash hands.
- Help the person into a comfortable position, either lying or sitting, with the back well supported so that the position can be maintained for a few minutes.
- Help the person to adjust or remove clothing to expose one axilla.
- Dry the skin of the axilla with a tissue – a film of moisture between the skin and the thermometer can cause an inaccurate reading.
- Place the thermometer probe in the axilla where the skin surfaces will surround it to get an accurate measurement.
- Help the person to hold their arm across their chest to retain the thermometer in the correct position.
- Leave the thermometer in place as per the manufacturer's instructions.
- Remain with the person, if required, to offer reassurance or to ensure that the thermometer remains in the correct position.
- Remove the thermometer when the optimum time for accurate reading has been reached.
- Read the temperature measured by the thermometer.
- Ensure that the person is left feeling as comfortable as possible to reassure and reduce anxiety.
- Clean or dispose of equipment as appropriate.
- Wash hands.
- Accurately document the temperature reading.

## EAR CANAL: TYMPANIC THERMOMETER

- Wash hands.
- Help the person into a comfortable position, in order to gain safe access to the ear.
- Prepare the thermometer as per the manufacturer's instructions.
- Apply a disposable sleeve to the thermometer.
- Switch the device on to ensure that it is calibrated and ready to take an accurate measurement.
- Stabilise the person's head to ensure the safe introduction of the thermometer probe.

- Align the probe tip with the ear canal and gently advance into the ear canal until the probe lightly seals the opening, ensuring a snug fit.
- Press and release the SCAN button.
- Remove the thermometer and dispose of the cover.
- Wash hands.
- Accurately document the temperature reading.

### EMPATHIC BEHAVIOUR

- Make sure that the person has not recently had a hot bath or been engaged in strenuous exercise as these will cause a temporary rise in body temperature.
- Always wash hands before and after carrying out the procedure.
- Explain the procedure in understandable terms to the patient to gain consent and co-operation and to encourage participation in care.
- When using a tympanic thermometer, remember to warn the person in advance that the probe will be inserted into the ear and that the thermometer will make a beeping noise.
- Ensure the patient's privacy and dignity is maintained during the procedure.
- Remember to offer some reassurance when you have read the measurement. Silence may be interpreted as an indication that something is wrong. 'That's normal' or 'That's grand' can be very reassuring to hear when you are worried about your condition.
- Remember, empathy is all about putting yourself in the patient's shoes and imagining what they are experiencing.

*The nurse didn't say anything after she took my temperature, but she was writing on the chart... There must be something wrong.*

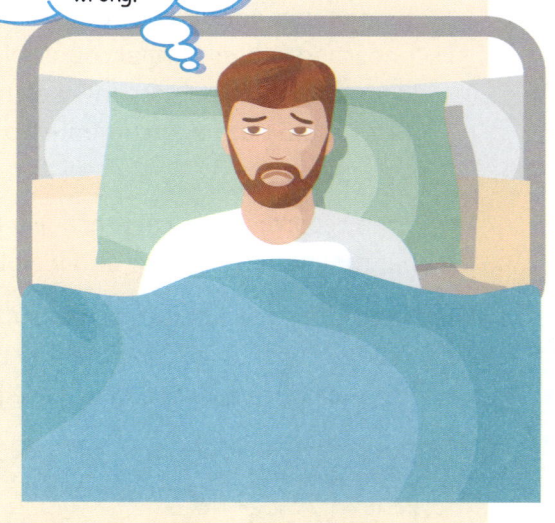

## RECORDING

Physiological observations are recorded graphically as this method is quicker and easier to read. Trends, e.g. an increasingly high temperature reading, can be detected promptly when recorded on a graph.

The patient's chart must always be checked at each entry. Three uniquely identifying pieces of information must be displayed on the chart: the person's name, date of birth and record number. In emergency situations, where any of these pieces of information cannot be obtained, the person's address may substitute for the missing information.

* Date and time is recorded each time a set of observations are measured.

* Times should always use the twenty-four-hour clock.

* Observations should be charted immediately as they may be forgotten or errors may be made if recorded at a later time.

* The nurse recording the information must sign or initial the entry. This ensures that enquiries about changes, etc. can be directed to the nurse concerned. Nurses are accountable for their actions and signing all documentation is an essential element of this aspect of the nurse's role. Care should not be documented on behalf of another nurse or healthcare professional.

* When recording clinical practice it is the writer's responsibility to ensure that their writing is clear and legible.

When recording a temperature measurement, it is recorded graphically on the observation chart using a single dot in the centre of the column. Dots from previous and subsequent readings are joined together using trend lines.

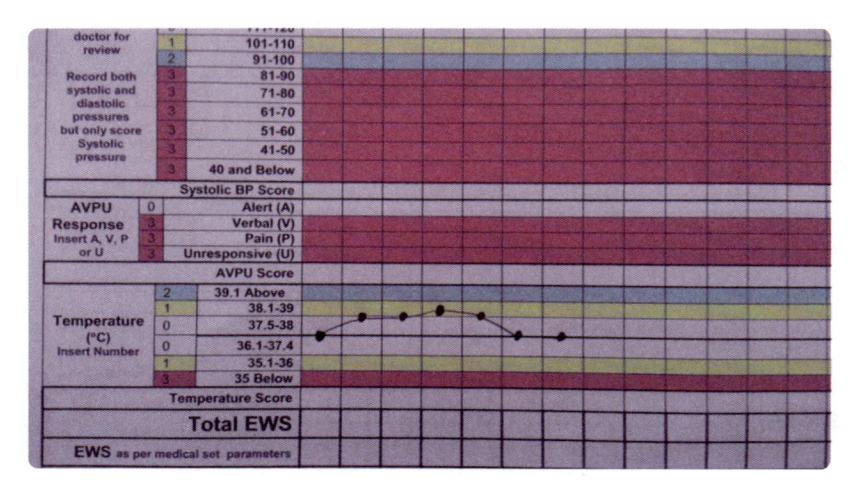

# Measuring and recording a pulse

### DEFINITION
A **pulse** is the rhythmic expansion and recoil of the elastic arteries caused by the ejection of blood from the left ventricle of the heart. As blood is ejected into the aorta a wave of contraction passes throughout the arteries. It can be palpated where an artery near the body surface can be pressed against a firm structure such as a bone.

Information that may be obtained from the pulse includes:

- the rate at which the heart is beating
- the rhythm or regularity of the heartbeat – the intervals between beats should be equal. Where they are not equal, this is described as being an irregular rhythm.
- the volume or strength of the beat – this gives an indication of the blood pressure and the state of the vessel wall (Grant & Waugh 2018).

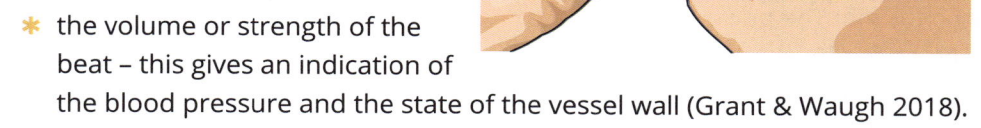

Normal pulse rates:

- Adult: 55–90 beats per minute
- Child: 70–110 beats per minute
- Baby: 80–160 beats per minute.

In adults:

- a pulse rate over 100 beats per minute is known as **tachycardia**
- a pulse rate below 60 beats per minute is known as **bradycardia**.

## WHY DO WE MEASURE PULSE?

- To ascertain a baseline pulse rate, rhythm and strength so that comparisons can be made

- To ascertain whether or not a person's pulse is within the normal range for their age
- Post-operatively, as an indication of the person's cardiovascular stability
- Post-operatively, as an indication of blood or fluid loss
- To evaluate the effect of treatments on someone with cardiovascular or pulmonary disease
- To monitor a person who is receiving a blood transfusion
- To assess for hydration status.

## MEASURING THE PULSE

The pulse can be located at several points on the body. The most common point to measure the pulse is the **radial pulse**. An easy way to remember the location of the radial pulse is to follow down the line of the thumb. The pulse can be felt by placing the tips of your first two fingers along the artery and applying light pressure until you feel the pulse. The rate can be counted using a watch with a second hand, for one full minute.

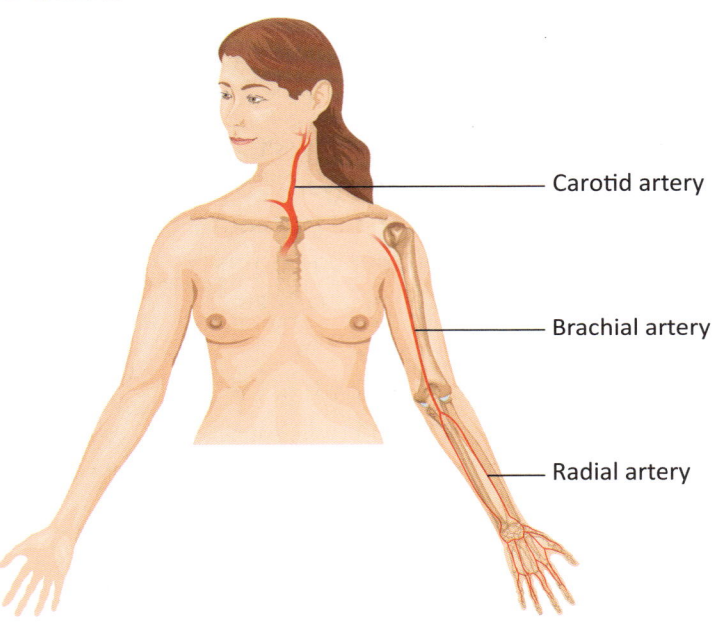

The **carotid pulse** can be located by running the fingers down the side of the larynx and applying gentle pressure to the carotid artery.

The **brachial pulse** can be located on the anterior aspect of the elbow by applying gentle pressure to the brachial artery.

- When taking a person's pulse, you need to ensure that they are sitting or lying in a comfortable position and are relaxed.
- Ideally the person should refrain from physical activity for twenty minutes prior to measuring the pulse.

* To obtain an accurate pulse rate, you must count the number of beats that you can feel in one full minute.

* In an emergency situation, the pulse rate can be counted for thirty seconds and multiplied by two to get the rate per minute.

* When undertaking a manual pulse, check other characteristics as well as the rate, e.g. rhythm and strength.

> ### EMPATHIC BEHAVIOUR
>
> * Always wash hands before carrying out the procedure.
>
> * Explain the procedure in understandable terms to the person to gain consent and co-operation and to encourage participation in care.
>
> * Ensure the person's privacy and dignity are maintained during the procedure.
>
> * Remember to be gentle but firm and confident when touching people directly. Gentleness sends a message of care and regard for the person. Firmness indicates confidence on the part of the nurse.
>
> * When the measurement has been taken, a reassuring comment will help prevent the person feeling stressed.

## RECORDING

Once the pulse rate has been obtained it should be recorded accurately. The rate is recorded graphically on the observation chart using a single dot in the centre of the column. Dots from previous and subsequent readings are joined together using trend lines.

Some observation sheets also provide a box to record information about the rhythm and the strength of the pulse.

# Measuring and recording respiration

> **DEFINITION**
>
> **Respiration –** the basic activity of the respiratory system is to supply sufficient oxygen for the body's metabolic needs and to remove carbon dioxide.
>
> Each breath consists of three phases: inspiration; expiration; pause.

## BREATHING ASSESSMENT

It is important to assess whether there is any obstruction to the person's airway from vomit, foreign bodies or the person's tongue.

Observe the person and the way they are breathing, including:

* the colour of their skin and mucous membranes (cyanosis is a blue tone to the skin and mucous membranes)
* any use of accessory muscles
* the rate, rhythm and depth of respiration
* shape and expansion of the chest.

Respiration may be assessed for the following reasons:

* To obtain a baseline measurement so that any alteration in the patient's breathing pattern can be promptly noticed
* To monitor a person who has breathing problems
* To help evaluate the effect of treatments on someone who has pulmonary disease.

The normal respiration rate is 12–18 breaths per minute. Respiration rates should be assessed over sixty seconds.

## ABNORMALITIES IN BREATHING

* **Dyspnoea –** the individual is conscious of the effort to breathe and finds it difficult.
* **Bradypnoea –** breathing that is slower than the normal rate.
* **Tachypnoea –** breathing that is faster than the normal rate and is shallow.
* **Apnoea –** a temporary cessation of breathing.

## MEASURING RESPIRATION RATE

This assessment is best carried out without the person's knowledge.

* Ensure correct positioning of the person in an upright position.
* Ensure that the person has rested for the previous five minutes.
* This measurement is usually taken directly after the pulse has been measured, with the person remaining in the same position.
* Count the respirations for sixty seconds by observing the rise and fall of the chest – this is the rate.
* Observe the depth and pattern of breathing and whether the breathing is through the nose or the mouth.

### EMPATHIC BEHAVIOUR

This is the one procedure that goes unexplained to the person. Knowing that the nurse is measuring the respiration rate will probably change the rate of breathing. The nurse remains as if still measuring the pulse but observes the fall and rise of the chest instead.

## RECORDING RESPIRATION RATE

Respiration rate is recorded graphically on the observation chart using a single dot in the centre of the column. Dots from previous and subsequent readings are joined together using trend lines.

# Pulse oximetry

Pulse oximetry is the non-invasive measurement of the oxygen saturation from haemoglobin in the arterial blood (Dougherty *et al.* 2015). It also provides information about the heart rate. A normal oxygen saturation will range between 95 per cent and 100 per cent. It is a useful tool in the assessment of respiratory status.

Pulse oximetry can be used as well as or instead of manual pulse rate measurement.

## EQUIPMENT

A pulse oximeter is a device that measures the amount of haemoglobin saturation in the tissue capillaries. The probe consists of two light-emitting diodes (LEDs) on one side of the probe and a photodetector on the other side. The device projects light through the tissues and measures the percentage of oxygen present.

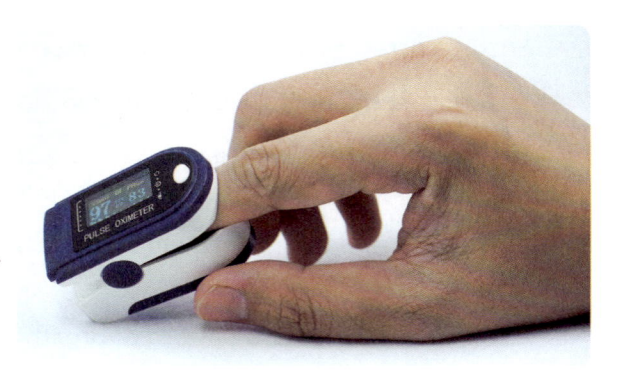

There are a variety of probes that are designed to fit suitable sites of the body that have an adequate pulsating tissue bed, e.g. the fingertip, earlobe, nose or toes.

The manufacturer's instructions should be followed when using this device.

The digital display on the pulse oximeter will indicate pulse rate and $SpO_2$ (oxygen saturation).

## MEASURING SATURATION LEVELS

An opportune time to carry out pulse oximetry is at the same time as the person's manual pulse rate and respirations are being measured. The person will already be in an appropriate position and will not have engaged in any physically strenuous exercise beforehand.

> **EMPATHIC BEHAVIOUR**
>
> * Carrying this out at the same time as manually measuring pulse and respiration will reduce the amount of disruption to the person's routine.
>
> * Explain the procedure in understandable terms to the person to gain consent and co-operation and to encourage participation in care.
>
> * Ensure the person's privacy and dignity are maintained during the procedure.
>
> * When the measurement has been taken, a reassuring comment will help prevent the person feeling stressed.

# Measuring and recording blood pressure

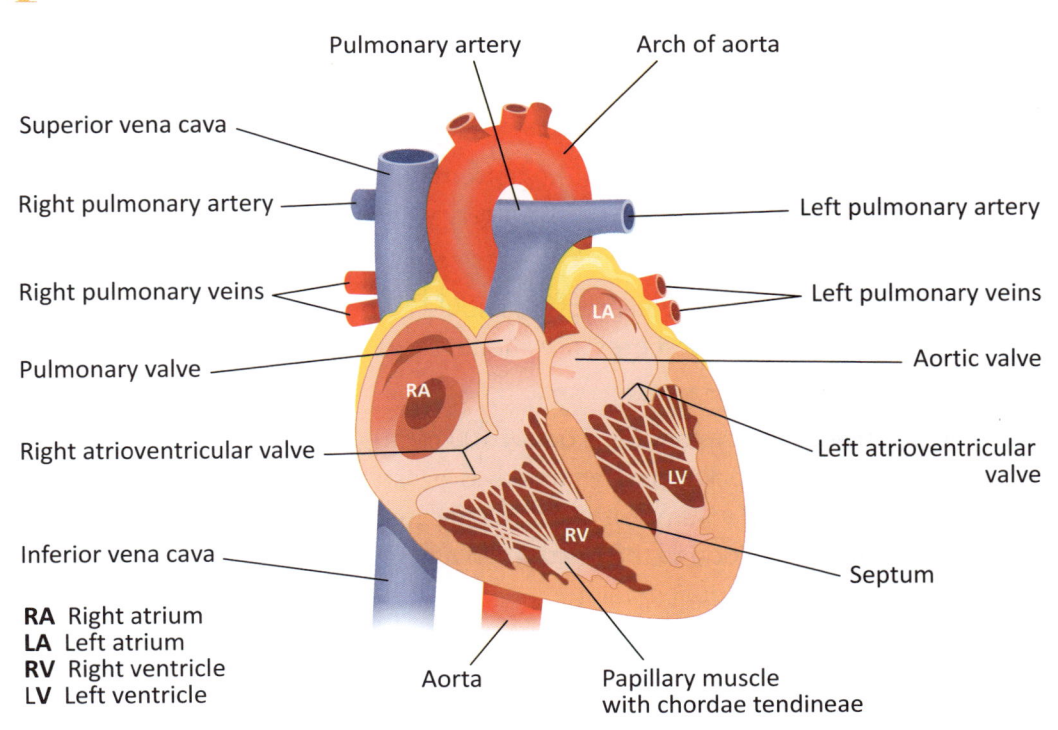

Pulmonary artery
Arch of aorta
Superior vena cava
Right pulmonary artery
Left pulmonary artery
Right pulmonary veins
Left pulmonary veins
Pulmonary valve
Aortic valve
Right atrioventricular valve
Left atrioventricular valve
Inferior vena cava
Septum
Aorta
Papillary muscle with chordae tendineae

**RA** Right atrium
**LA** Left atrium
**RV** Right ventricle
**LV** Left ventricle

## DEFINITION

**Blood pressure** is the force or pressure that the blood exerts on the walls of the blood vessels. The systemic arterial blood pressure is the result of discharge of blood from the left ventricle of the heart into the already full aorta (Grant & Waugh 2018).

## Exercise

Revise the cardiac cycle in your Anatomy and Physiology module so that you have a full understanding of the physiology of blood pressure.

## NORMAL, LOW AND HIGH BLOOD PRESSURE

Blood pressure can fluctuate within a wide range and still be considered as being within normal limits.

Blood pressure is expressed as a fraction or a ratio, e.g. 120/80. The top number indicates **systolic** pressure, which is the pressure in the artery when the heart is contracting (systole). The bottom number indicates **diastolic** pressure, which is the pressure in the artery when the heart is at rest (diastole).

At rest, normal systolic blood pressure should be between 110 and 140 mmHg. Diastolic blood pressure should be between 70 and 80 mmHg (Grant & Waugh 2018).

In **hypotension** the systolic BP is below 100 mmHg. Hypotension can be the first indication of shock (where vital body processes shut down in response to a reduction in blood volume). It can also indicate that there is not sufficient pressure to pump blood to the head when a person is standing or sitting, and it can cause the individual to faint.

**Hypertension** is an elevation of the blood pressure and may be acute or chronic. A reading of above 140/90 is defined as hypertension. The measurement is based not on one reading but on three or more readings taken at rest, several days apart. Hypertension increases the risk of having a stroke or heart attack.

## FACTORS AFFECTING BLOOD PRESSURE READINGS

* **Blood volume** – reductions in blood volume caused by dehydration or blood loss can cause a drop in blood pressure.
* **Elasticity of the artery walls** – This can be affected by atherosclerosis (a build-up of fat deposits in the blood vessels).
* **Nicotine** – a vasoconstrictor that can increase blood pressure.
* **Age** – BP increases with age.
* **Gender** – Men generally have a higher BP than women.
* **Weight** – Higher weight tends to increase BP.
* **Emotional factors** – Stress, fear, anxiety and excitement tend to increase BP.
* **Diet** – A high salt intake can increase BP.
* **Time of day** – BP tends to be higher later in the day.
* **White coat hypertension** – related to the anxiety experienced when in a medical environment.
* **Gravity** – If an individual stands up quickly from a lying position the BP may fall; this is known as orthostatic hypotension.
* **Family history** related to coronary heart disease.
* **Sleep** – BP is lowest when sleeping.

## WHY DO WE MEASURE BLOOD PRESSURE?

* To obtain a baseline reading (a reading taken as a reference for future readings)
* As a measure of cardiovascular function
* To screen patients for underlying disease or complications
* Post-operatively, as an indication of blood or fluid loss
* To ascertain whether a person's blood pressure is within the normal range for their age.

## TAKING BLOOD PRESSURE

### EQUIPMENT

Blood pressure is taken with a manual sphygmomanometer and a stethoscope, or with a fully automatic machine.

A sphygmomanometer consists of a rubber cuff connected to a rubber bulb used to inflate the cuff and a meter that registers the pressure in the cuff. It is essential that the correct size of the cuff be used to ensure accuracy of the BP reading. When the bulb is pumped, air is forced into the rubber bladder within the cuff, and to deflate the cuff there is a release valve. The stethoscope should be placed over the brachial artery at the antecubital fossa (inside of the elbow). The person's arm should be free from clothing, supported and placed at heart level. Legs should be uncrossed with feet flat on the floor.

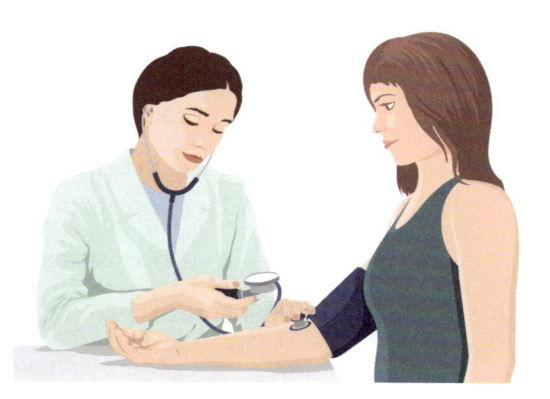

### PROCEDURE

* Wrap the cuff of the sphygmomanometer around the arm, with the bladder centred over the artery and above the elbow. The lower edge of the cuff should be 2–3 cm above the brachial artery pulsation.
* Palpate the brachial artery while pumping air into the cuff. When the pulse can no longer be felt, rapidly inflate the cuff for a further 20–30 mmHg.
* Deflate the cuff. The point at which the pulse reappears approximates the systolic blood pressure.
* Deflate the cuff completely and wait for thirty seconds.
* The stethoscope should be firmly, but without too much pressure, placed on the brachial artery where the brachial pulse is palpable.
* Inflate the cuff again to 20–30 mmHg above the predicted systolic blood pressure.
* Release the cuff slowly until the first tapping sounds are heard (Korotkoff sounds). This is the systolic blood pressure. Continue to slowly release the air, listening to the Korotkoff sounds. The point at which the sounds disappear is the best representation of the diastolic blood pressure.
* Continue to deflate the cuff until you are sure the sounds have disappeared.

> ## EMPATHIC BEHAVIOUR
>
> * Always wash hands before carrying out the procedure.
>
> * Explain the procedure in understandable terms to the person to gain consent and co-operation, and to encourage participation in care.
>
> * Ensure that you maintain the person's privacy and dignity throughout the procedure; they may have to remove some outer clothing so that you can access the arm.
>
> * It is important to explain that the cuff will become quite tight and may be uncomfortable. Reassuring the person that this will only be momentary will help to reduce any fear or anxiety that they may have.
>
> * Remember to be gentle but firm and confident when touching people directly. Gentleness gives a message of care and regard for the person. Firmness indicates confidence on the part of the nurse.
>
> * When the measurement has been taken, a reassuring comment will help prevent the person feeling stressed.

## RECORDING BLOOD PRESSURE READINGS

Once the systolic and diastolic BP values have been obtained, they should be recorded accurately.

Charting on an observation chart takes the form of a graph. The systolic pressure is marked by an arrow at the top and the diastolic value by an arrow at the bottom. The space between the readings is drawn in either a dotted or a continuous line.

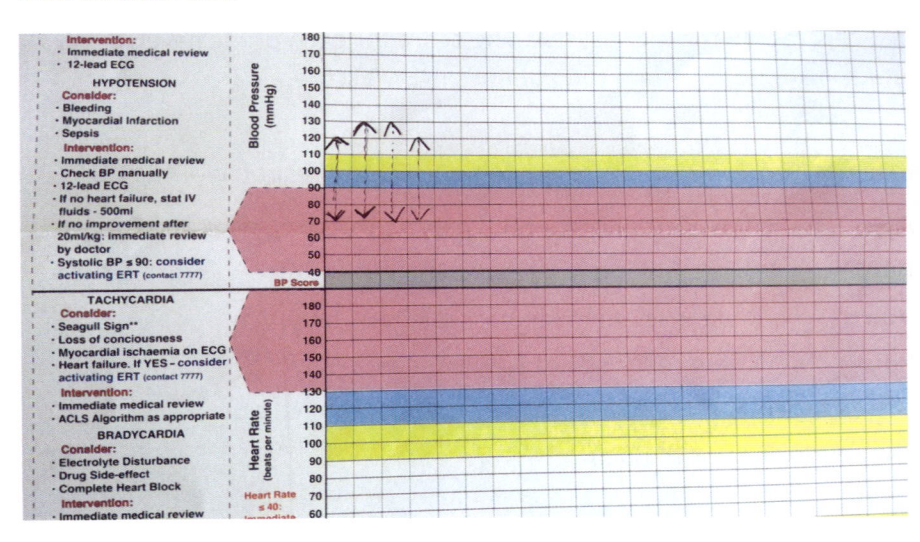

# Early warning system (EWS)

Early warning systems help healthcare staff recognise and respond to clinical deterioration. They are used in hospitals in Australia, America and Europe. The Irish system is known as INEWS (Irish National Early Warning System). It is a bedside score and track and trigger system which staff calculate from routinely collected physiological observations: pulse rate, respiration rate, blood pressure reading, pulse oximetry, temperature.

This system enables nurses and medical staff to anticipate and recognise deterioration in a person's condition, to escalate the actions needed to be taken in response to the person's changing condition and to continually evaluate the person's condition.

When physiological observations are measured, they are recorded on an INEWS chart. These observations are:

* respiratory rate
* $SpO_2$
* $FiO_2$ (room air or supplemental oxygen)
* heart rate
* blood pressure
* neurological response or ACVPU (see below)
* temperature.

INEWS allocates 0–3 points to measurements of each of these seven physiological parameters, where a score of 0 represents the least risk and a score of 3 represents the highest risk. The score for each of the seven INEWS parameters is added to obtain the patient's INEWS score.

> Disability on the INEWS chart refers to neurological response – **ACVPU**.
> * **Alert** – Patient is alert and oriented to person, place, time and event.
> * **Confused** – New confusion or altered mental status.
> * **Voice** – The patient responds to verbal stimuli only.
> * **Pain** – The patient responds to painful stimuli only.
> * **Unresponsive** – The patient does not respond to stimuli.
>
> (See Appendix 3 INEWS Chart)

INEWS aims to identify early signs of a patient's deterioration. The inbuilt escalation protocol prompts more timely medical review and treatment of patients. For example, occurrence of sepsis is considered if there is an INEWS score of 4 or higher (5 or higher if the patient is on oxygen) and a suspicion of infection.

### Sepsis

Sepsis is a potentially life-threatening complication of an infection. The most effective way to reduce mortality from sepsis is through early recognition and treatment. The INEWS chart facilitates the early recognition of the signs of sepsis in acute hospital settings.

### Exercise

For each of the observations, ensure that you understand the theory behind their measurement.

Practise each measurement, and be sure to include the empathic behaviour that is required for each.

Practise recording the measurements on the INEWS chart in Appendix 3.

When you are competent in each observation, carry out the measurement and recording of a full set of observations on one of your classmates.

# 11

# Ethics and Codes of Professional Conduct

In this chapter you will learn about:

- Ethics for nurses
- The ethical principles that guide nursing practice: autonomy, beneficence, non-maleficence, confidentiality and consent
- Codes of nursing ethics
- Values in nursing and midwifery

## What is ethics?

### DEFINITION

**Ethics** is about right and wrong. Ethics is a set of moral principles that govern behaviours, thoughts and actions. As individuals, our moral principles are based on our own personal beliefs and value systems. Our belief systems are strongly influenced by what we learn from our parents and from our culture and the society that we are part of.

In the context of nursing, ethics is about making decisions in relation to what a nurse ought to do or should do in his/her practice. It is underpinned by professional values and beliefs. In professions, values, beliefs and accepted behaviours are expressed as codes of conduct (NMBI 2014).

Ethical principles incorporate the values, beliefs and standards that guide professional practice. The ethical principles that guide nursing practice are autonomy, beneficence, non-maleficence, confidentiality and consent.

## AUTONOMY

Autonomy involves self-determination and self-authorship. It is the freedom of each individual to make their own life choices. In western cultures, like Ireland's, individual choice is highly valued. In some other cultures, e.g. in South Asia, family and communal decision-making is considered more important than individual decision-making.

Two philosophers, Immanuel Kant (1724–1804) and John Stuart Mill (1806–1873), have greatly influenced the way in which we understand what respect for autonomy includes.

Both say that every person has unconditional worth and should be valued. Kant believed this worth was due to our ability, as humans, to have free will that we can follow independently. Mill believed that each person is worthy of respect because of their unique individuality. In the context of modern living, an autonomous person is someone who is capable of making important decisions about their own lives on the basis of their own beliefs and values. Because of the significance attached to autonomy in western cultures, respect for autonomous choice is considered an important moral and legal right (Dooley & McCarthy 2012).

* **Negative autonomy** is the person's right to refuse treatment.
* **Positive autonomy** is the person's right to be facilitated, as much as possible, to make decisions about the type of care and treatment they want.

Truth telling, which is a fundamental moral value in nursing, is based on respect for autonomy. There is a moral obligation on a nurse to be truthful in their conversations with the people they provide care for, and this requires skilful communication. In situations where people ask not to be told the truth of their condition, this does not justify lying to them or misleading them.

## BENEFICENCE

Beneficence is the act of doing something for the benefit of another person. In nursing practice, it means that the nurse always acts for the benefit of the patient. Nursing, as a profession, is considered to be altruistic, which means that nurses are willing to work for the advantage of others, i.e. patients. In adhering to this moral principle, nurses promote the health and wellbeing of those they care for.

## NON-MALEFICENCE

Non-maleficence is the principle of avoiding harm. Nurses are required to prevent and remove the conditions that cause harm and, in doing so, to promote good.

It is connected with **justice**, which is about veracity (truth) and fairness. Nurses are non-judgmental and treat all patients equally. When applying the nursing process to provide care for a person, the nurse's ultimate goal is to meet the person's needs and ensure their wellbeing. This is unconditional, and a fundamental part of being a nurse is having unconditional regard for the person who is being cared for. This can be challenging, particularly when resources are scarce, and nurses endeavour to utilise and distribute those resources fairly. There is no room for bias or prejudice in nursing practice.

## CONFIDENTIALITY

Nurses must respect the confidences that a patient shares with them, as well as keeping patient information confidential.

Confidentiality expresses respect for autonomy and privacy. It enables patients to be open about personal issues, concerns and questions. It is an implicit part of the nurse–patient relationship and forms the basis of a therapeutic relationship built on trust and respect. In healthcare generally, including nursing, there is a presumed right of confidentiality on the patient's part.

However, sometimes serious extenuating circumstances may call for the principle to be qualified to some degree. On some occasions the nurse may be legally obliged to disclose private information about a person or their condition. It may be necessary in some instances to protect the interests of the patient or perhaps the interests of others in society. Sometimes the safety of the patient or of others is justification for breaching confidentiality. These situations can be complex and cause ethical dilemmas for nurses. Other ethical principles will be considered simultaneously, and the nurse must use their professional judgment to decide the best thing to do in that particular situation. Remember that ethics is all about trying to do the right thing.

## CONSENT

Prior to undergoing any kind of nursing or medical procedure, the person must consent to it. This is an absolute ethical and legal requirement. In order to give consent, a person must be fully informed in relation to all aspects of the pending procedure. When the person has full understanding, they are in a better position to decide whether or not to consent. The requirement of **informed consent** ensures that the principles of autonomy, beneficence and non-maleficence are respected. Gaining informed consent before carrying out a procedure is a means of respecting a patient's privacy and dignity.

Providing information in a way that is understandable to the person requires the nurse to have empathy for that person and it is facilitated through open and honest communication. Adequate communication requires listening as well as speaking. The person needs to be informed about the potential advantages and disadvantages of any proposed treatment and alternatives to treatment, in order for them to reflect and deliberate on whether or not to accept the treatment being offered.

# Codes of nursing ethics

An international code of ethics for nurses was first adopted by the International Council of Nurses (ICN) in 1953. It was most recently revised in 2012 (ICN 2012).

The ICN states that nurses have four fundamental responsibilities: to promote health; to prevent illness; to restore health; and to alleviate suffering.

It believes that the need for nursing is universal and that inherent in nursing is a respect for human rights, including cultural rights, the right to life and choice, to dignity and to be treated with respect. Nursing care is respectful of and unrestricted by considerations of age, colour, creed, culture, disability or illness, gender, sexual orientation, nationality, politics, race or social status. Nurses provide care and support to the individual, the family and the community and coordinate their services with those of related groups.

The *ICN Code of Ethics for Nurses* is a guide for nursing practice based on social values and needs and it is intended to be applied to the realities of nursing and healthcare in changing societies. The code gives a framework for the development of codes of conduct and is used by nursing regulatory bodies in individual countries.

Ireland's most recent *Code of Professional Conduct and Ethics for Registered Nurses and Midwives* was published in 2014 (NMBI 2014). The purpose of the code is to guide nurses and midwives in their day-to-day practice and help them to understand their professional responsibilities in caring for patients in a safe, ethical and effective way within the Irish legal and regulatory framework.

It aims to:

* support and guide nurses and midwives in their ethical and clinical decision-making, their ongoing reflection and professional self-development
* inform the general public about the professional care they can expect from nurses and midwives
* emphasise the importance of the obligation of nurses and midwives to recognise and respond to the needs of patients and families
* set standards for the regulation, monitoring and enforcement of professional conduct.

All registered nurses and midwives should adhere to the code's principles, values and standards of conduct. Every nurse and midwife has a responsibility to uphold the values of their profession to ensure their practice reflects high standards of professional practice and protects the public. If a registered nurse or midwife does not follow the code and a complaint is made against them, the NMBI can investigate that nurse or midwife.

The Nurses and Midwives Act 2011 requires the NMBI to provide guidelines to the schools of nursing and midwifery on ethical standards and behaviours for students. Nursing and midwifery students should become familiar with the code as part of their education.

The code is based on five principles. They govern:

1. Respect for dignity of the person
2. Professional responsibility and accountability
3. Quality of practice
4. Trust and confidentiality
5. Collaboration with others.

(In Chapter 12, Medication Management, you will see how each of the five principles is applied to nursing practice.)

Each principle underpins the code's ethical values and related standards of conduct and practice and guides the relationships between nurses, midwives, patients and colleagues. The ethical values state the primary goals and obligations of nurses and midwives. The standards of conduct and professional practice follow on from these values and show the attitudes and behaviours that members of the public have the right to expect from nurses and midwives. The trio of principles, values and standards of conduct are of equal importance and should be considered in association with each other (NMBI 2014).

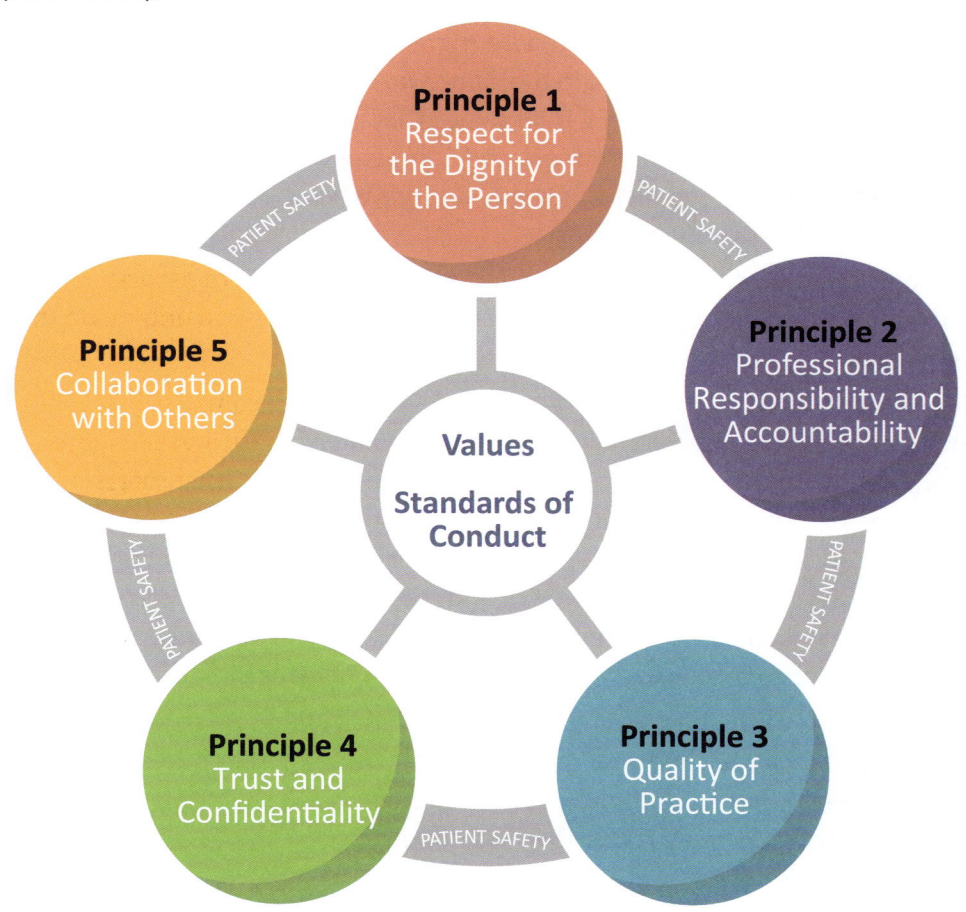

**Principle 1** Respect for the Dignity of the Person

**Principle 2** Professional Responsibility and Accountability

**Principle 3** Quality of Practice

**Principle 4** Trust and Confidentiality

**Principle 5** Collaboration with Others

Values
Standards of Conduct

PATIENT SAFETY

Source: NMBI (2014:10) Code of Professional Conduct and Ethics for Registered Nurses and Registered Midwives

> **Exercise**
>
> Download the *Code of Professional Conduct and Ethics* from the Nursing and Midwifery Board of Ireland website (www.nmbi.ie/Standards-Guidance/Code). For each of the five principles, read the Values, the Standards of Conduct and the Supporting Guidance.

# Values in nursing and midwifery

Our values and what we believe in determine our behaviours. We all have our individual and personal beliefs. In the same way, nursing as a profession has its own beliefs and values and it is its values that guide nursing and midwifery practice. Care, compassion, kindness and competence are values that are considered synonymous with nursing and this is what the general public expect from nurses and midwives.

However, in Ireland, a number of incidents occurred that were associated with nursing and midwifery practice that challenged this perception and made the general public question what nurses and midwives value.

These incidents made it necessary for the government to commission investigations, and the reports published as a result of these investigations prompted nursing leaders to question the current values in the professions. The three organisations that lead and support nurses – the Office of the Chief Nursing Officer in the Department of Health, the Office of the Nursing and Midwifery Services Director in the HSE and the Nursing and Midwifery Board of Ireland – collaborated with each other to come up with a way to explore and reaffirm the core principles that guide nursing practice in Ireland today.

They agreed that the best way to do this was to talk and listen to nurses and midwives themselves, and so a consultative process was set up to do exactly that. Nationally, nurses and midwives were asked to reflect on the reasons why they became nurses and midwives and to identify what was important to them in the provision of care and what it is that they value as professionals. This extensive consultation identified and agreed that the three core values that underpin nursing and midwifery practice in modern-day Ireland are compassion, care and commitment.

The Office of the Chief Nursing Officer in the Department of Health subsequently published a position paper outlining actions that are needed to continuously nurture these values in practice (DoH 2016). As we discussed in Chapter 1, nursing has its basis in science. Nursing practice is underpinned by a body of knowledge that has been generated from research, but this knowledge will only be of benefit to patients if nurses are competent in applying it in practice. This is the art of nursing.

The position paper outlines how these core values can be embedded into nursing and midwifery practice in the provision of good-quality, safe care. This is the responsibility of each individual nurse and it is the responsibility of the structures that guide and support practice to facilitate it.

**Managerial systems – develop supports where values thrive in practice**

**DOH HSE NMBI**

**Culture – create a culture for learning and developing values in practice**

**People in the health service – support the expression of values as behaviour**

### Exercise

In groups, discuss each of the following principles individually and what it means in the context of patient care. Make a poster for each principle with pictures and words that represent what they mean:

* Autonomy
* Beneficence
* Non-maleficence
* Justice
* Confidentiality
* Consent

# Medication Management

In this chapter you will learn about:

* The importance of precision in administering drugs
* The personnel qualified to prescribe and administer drugs
* A range of drug preparations
* The routes of drug administration
* The importance of following the correct procedure in relation to checking the prescription, patient identity, medication, dosage, route and time of administration
* How the administration of a drug is recorded

## Introduction

> **DEFINITIONS**
>
> A **medicine** is 'any substance or combination of substances presented as having properties for treating or preventing disease in human beings' (Dougherty *et al.* 2015).
>
> **Medication management** is 'The safe, technically effective and economic use of medicines to ensure that people using health and social services get the maximum benefit from the medicines they need while at the same time minimizing potential harm' (HIQA 2014).

Medication management is a fundamental part of the nursing role and it requires a high level of skill and accuracy. Nurses administer many different types of medication using many different methods of administration. The potential for error is always present and the consequences of making a mistake when dealing with medicines range from minor to fatal.

The prescribing, dispensing, supply and administration of medicines in Ireland is regulated to protect the public and to aid patients in receiving effective and safe quality healthcare involving medicines. It is critical that nurses and midwives are fully aware of their responsibilities in relation to legislation, regulations and policies on medication management. The laws, regulations and policies provide legal direction and sound guidance to ensure that nurses ask correct and relevant questions and make the right decisions when managing medicines.

# Legislation

The legislation that governs the management of medicines in Ireland includes:

* Irish Medicines Board Acts 1995 and 2006
* Pharmacy Act 2007
* Misuse of Drugs Acts (MDA) 1977 and 1984
* Irish Medicines Board (Miscellaneous Provisions) Act 2006
* Misuse of Drugs (Amendment) Regulations (2007)
* Misuse of Drugs (Amendment) Regulations (2014).

### WHO CAN LEGALLY PRESCRIBE MEDICATION?

In Ireland, registered medical practitioners, registered dentists and registered nurse or midwife prescribers can prescribe medicines. Nurse prescribing was first introduced in Ireland in 2007 when new legislation was passed and a new division on the NMBI's register was created – registered nurse/midwife prescriber. Postgraduate education programmes were devised to equip nurses and midwives with the knowledge and skills to take on this expansion in practice. Nurses and midwives who undergo this training are granted the legal authority to prescribe within their scope of practice and are supported by guidance and regulation (NMBI 2019).

Registered pharmacists are responsible for dispensing medicines in Ireland. Their practice is directed by the Pharmacy Act 2007 and regulated by the Pharmaceutical Society of Ireland.

Where nurses have expanded their practice to prescribe, they have found that it has allowed them to provide more holistic care to patients and has provided them with greater job satisfaction as a result. They also found that it increased their levels of responsibility and accountability (Condell *et al.* 2014).

# Guidance on medication administration

The Nursing and Midwifery Board of Ireland, as the regulator of the nursing and midwifery professions, has developed guidance on medication administration (NMBI 2020). The NMBI's practice standards are based on the five principles of the *Code of Professional Conduct and Ethics for Registered Nurses and Registered Midwives* (NMBI 2014).

The HSE, in conjunction with the NMBI, has designed an e-learning programme that enables nurses to refresh their knowledge and skills and keep abreast of changes in legislation and practice. This e-learning programme must be undertaken at least every two years.

HIQA offers guidance on the medication needs of older people and children and adults with disabilities living in residential care (HIQA 2015). It also provides guidance on the accurate administration of medications when a person transfers between health and social care services (HIQA 2014).

> ### DEFINITIONS
>
> **Contraindication –** A specific situation in which a medicine should *not* be used because it might be harmful to the patient, perhaps because the patient is allergic to the drug or because it might interact with other medicines that they have taken.
>
> **Indication –** the indication for a drug refers to the use of that drug for treating a specific problem. A drug sometimes has more than one indication, which means that there is more than one disease for which it could be used.

**Interaction** – when a substance affects the activity of a drug when both are administered together.

**Pharmacology** – the study of drugs and the effects that they have on the human body.

**Polypharmacy** – the term used to describe taking different medicines; generally understood to be the concurrent use of multiple medicines by one individual. Polypharmacy is common in Ireland, with one in five people over the age of fifty years regularly taking five or more medicines and one in two people over seventy-five years regularly taking five or more medicines (TILDA 2012).

**Side effect** – an effect that occurs in addition to the intended primary effect of the drug. This can be harmful or unpleasant, or, in some cases, beneficial for the patient.

## ROUTES OF ADMINISTRATION AND DRUG PREPARATIONS

There is a wide variety of routes for administrating medications and a wide range of drug preparations. Some routes are more invasive than others. When prescribing a medication, the prescriber needs to look at the patient holistically and consider which is the most suitable route for administration for that individual and if the drug is available in that preparation form.

### ORAL (PO)

Oral medications (abbreviated to PO, from the Latin *per os* – 'by mouth') are taken by mouth. They are either swallowed by the patient or given through a feeding tube, e.g. a nasogastric (NG) tube or a percutaneous endoscopic gastrostomy (PEG) tube. This is the most convenient route for taking medications, and it is generally very safe and inexpensive.

However, it is not a safe route for patients who have a reduced level of consciousness as there is a risk of choking. Neither is it suitable when patients are feeling nauseated or are fasting.

Oral medications can come in tablet or capsule form or as liquids.

* A **tablet** is a compressed preparation that is swallowed. Some tablets have coatings that are resistant to gastric acids so that they disintegrate in the duodenum, jejunum or colon.

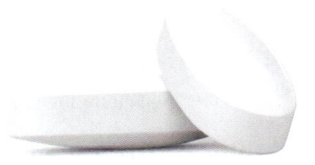

* A **capsule** has a gelatinous covering enclosing the active substance. These can be easier to swallow than tablets and are designed to remain intact for some hours after ingestion in order to delay absorption.

* **Liquid** drug preparations are easily swallowed and suitable for administration through NG and PEG tubes.

**Sublingual** (SL) medications are placed under the tongue and are absorbed by the mucous membranes. Absorption happens quickly, so it is a suitable method for administering emergency cardiac drugs.

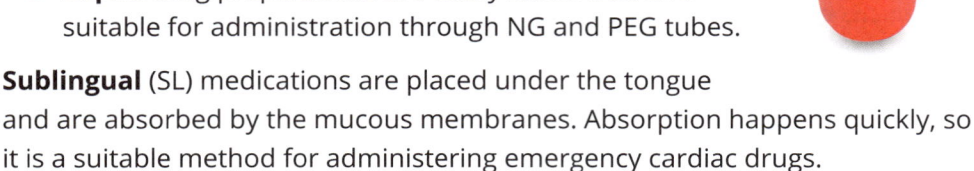

**Buccal** (BC) medications are placed in the mouth in the space between the gums and the cheek and are absorbed by the mucous membranes. Absorption happens quickly so it is a suitable method for administering drugs like anti-epilepsy drugs during a seizure.

## TOPICAL

These medications are applied onto the skin or mucous membranes usually for a localised effect, e.g. creams and ointments. Creams are emulsions of oil and water and are generally absorbed easily by the skin. Ointments are more greasy and are absorbed more slowly.

**Transdermal** (TD) medications are applied to the outermost layer of the skin, usually as a medicated patch or disc that allows the medication to be absorbed at a slow and constant rate, in order to produce a systemic effect.

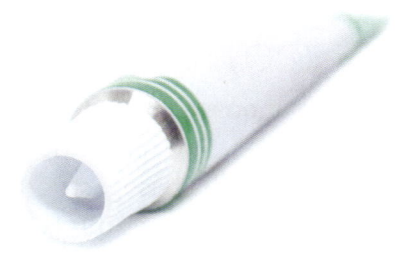

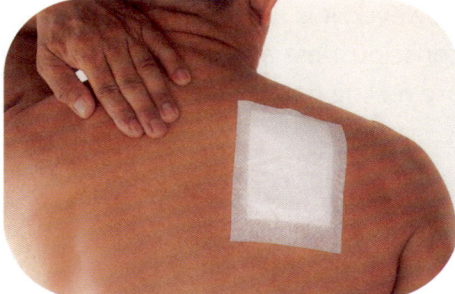

## RECTAL (PR)

Preparations that are administered via the rectum may exert a local effect on the mucosa of the large bowel (e.g. an anti-inflammatory effect in cases of ulcerative colitis) or a systemic effect (e.g. analgesic suppositories).

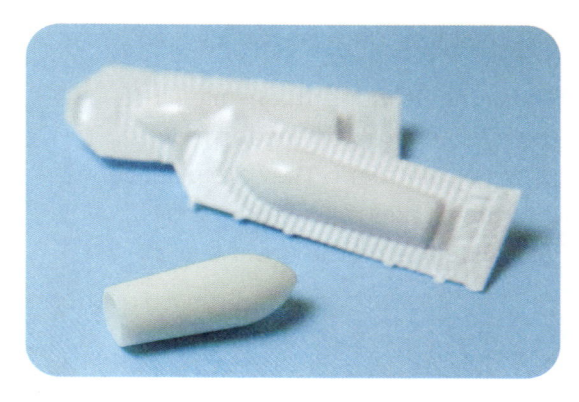

Rectal drug preparations include:

* suppositories that are inserted into the rectum
* micro-enemas and large-volume enemas.

## VAGINAL (PV)

These medications are inserted into the vaginal canal, usually for localised effect, e.g. pessaries that treat fungal infections.

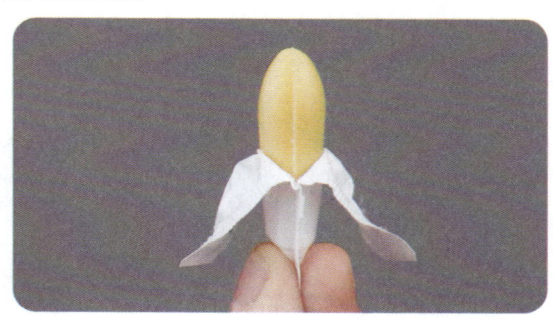

## PULMONARY

These are aerosols that are inhaled via the lungs. They are generally used to improve lung dilation or to help clear secretions that are congestive. Pulmonary drug preparations can be administered by inhalers or nebulisers.

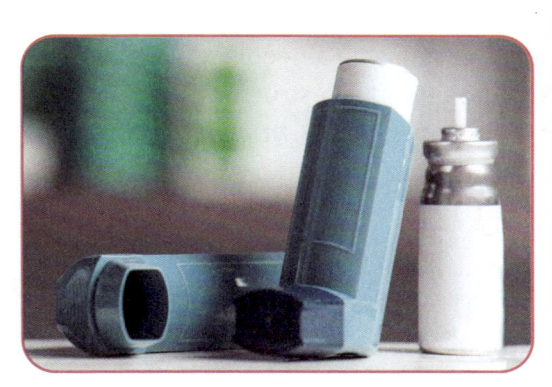

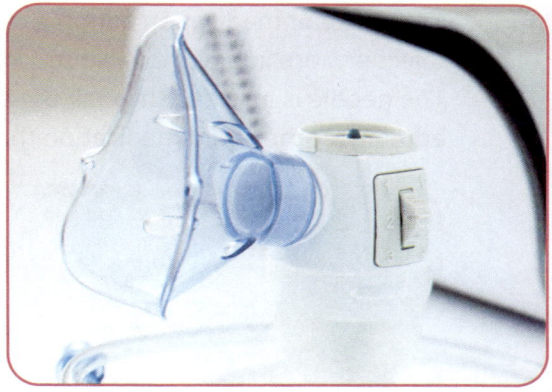

## OPTHALMIC

These medications are instilled into the eye, generally in the form of drops or ointment. They are instilled into the pocket that is formed by gently pulling on the lower eyelid.

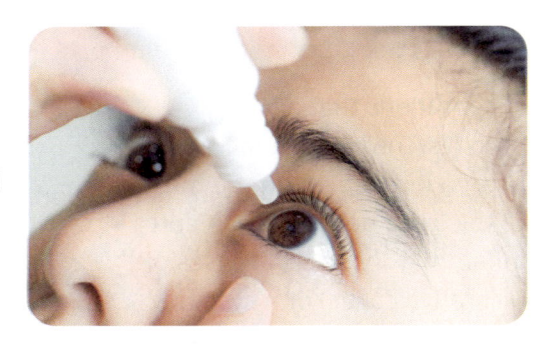

## NASAL

These are generally sprays or drops that are introduced into the nasal cavity. They may be used to relieve local symptoms such as allergic rhinitis or to allow the delivery of drugs systemically, e.g. drugs to treat migraine.

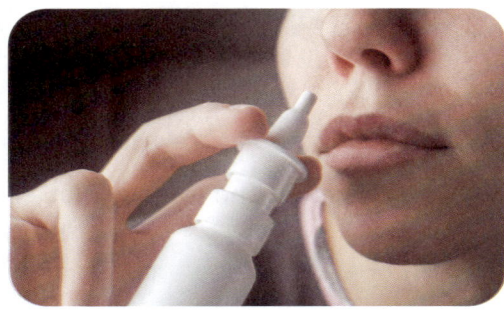

## OTIC

These medications are introduced into the ear for local effect, e.g. for softening ear wax or treating ear infections.

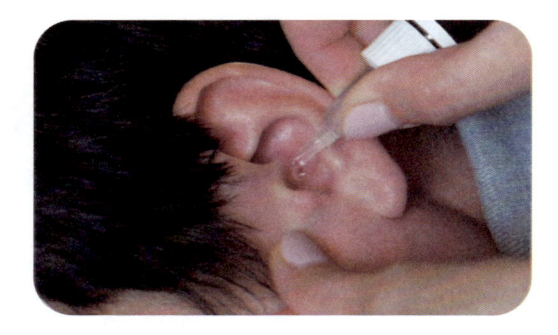

## INJECTIONS AND INFUSIONS

This route of medication administration is high on the scale of invasiveness. Injections are liquid preparations that are given using a needle and syringe. The needle is inserted through the skin into underlying structures to administer the liquid medication that is contained in the syringe.

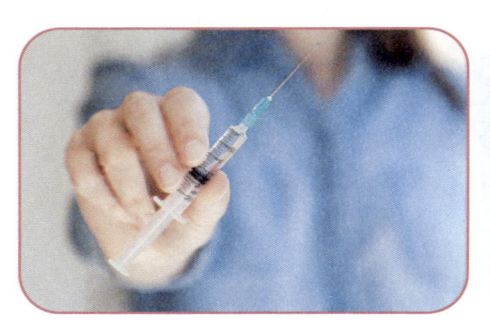

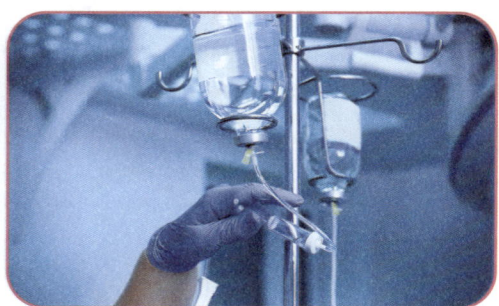

* **Injections** are small in volume.
* **Infusions** are larger volumes of fluid that can be given either intermittently or continuously.

There are different methods of injection:

* **Subcutaneous injection (SC)** – given beneath the epidermis into the loose fat and connective tissue beneath the dermis, e.g. small doses of non-irritating water-soluble substances such as insulin. Subcutaneous tissue does not have a rich blood supply, so the medications given are absorbed slowly by the body. A short fine needle is used for this method.

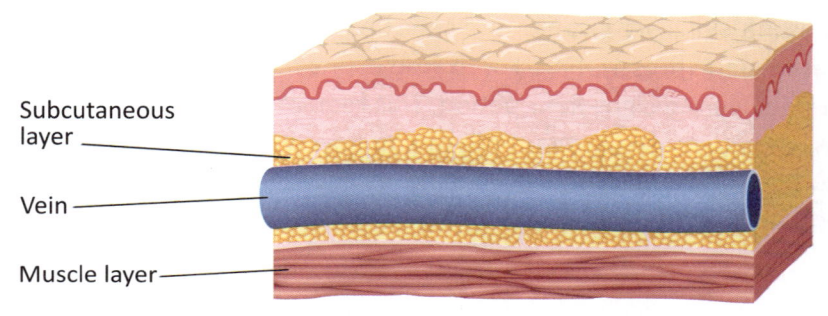

Subcutaneous layer
Vein
Muscle layer

* **Subcutaneous infusion** – continuous infusion of fluids or medication into the subcutaneous tissues. Fluids can be given to maintain hydration in patients with mild to moderate dehydration. Most commonly used with elderly patients or in palliative care.

* **Intramuscular injections (IM)** – deposits medication into deep muscle tissue, beneath the subcutaneous tissue. Muscles have a rich blood supply, so this facilitates the absorption of the medication. A longer needle than that required for subcutaneous injection is required here.

IM   IV   SC

* **Intravenous injections (IV)** – the introduction of medication or solutions directly into the circulatory system through a vein. A flexible plastic cannula is inserted into the vein using a sharp metal introducer. Once inserted, the introducer is removed and the cannula remains in the vein.

* **Intravenous infusion –** Fluids and medications can be given through this route at a constant rate over a prescribed time period, or given intermittently. This method allows the medication to be well diluted and less irritating to the vein while ensuring that the medication reaches the circulatory system without being altered in any way. It is a very effective and efficient method of drug administration.

## TIME AND FREQUENCY OF ADMINISTRATION

Precision and accuracy are essential in drug administration to ensure that the person taking the medicine gains maximum benefit from the drug prescribed. Intravenous infusions are given over a specified amount of time, which will be clearly stated in the prescription. For example: one litre of normal saline may be prescribed over an eight-hour period. This requires the nurse to calculate how much should infuse per hour; the rate of flow will have to be calculated to ensure accuracy. The ability to calculate doses and rates in drug administration is an important skill.

The prescriber of any medication must always clearly state the dose and frequency. There are accepted abbreviations, based on Latin, that are used in prescriptions. For example:

* **BD –** twice daily. This means twice in a twenty-four-hour period. It should be administered with twelve hours between doses.
* **TDS –** three times daily. This means three times in a twenty-four-hour period. It should be administered with eight hours between doses.
* **QDS –** four times daily. This means four times in a twenty-four-hour period. It should be administered with six hours between doses.
* **PRN –** as required. It may be given if necessary.
* **Mane –** given in the morning.
* **Nocte –** given at night.

# Safety in the administration of medications

Safety is the priority in all aspects of drug use, both prescribing and administration.

Guiding Principle 4 of the *Guidance for Registered Nurses and Midwives on Medication Administration* (NMBI 2020) outlines the ten rights of drug administration. This is a guide for nurses to ensure that medication errors are avoided, and that patient safety is protected

The ten rights of drug administration are as follows:

1. Right patient. Verify the identity of the patient to whom the medicine is being administered through the hospital wristband, photograph or name, hospital number and/or date of birth with the medicine chart.
2. Right reason. Understand the intended purpose of the medicines to be administered.
3. Right drug. Confirm that the name of the dispensed medicine to be administered corresponds with the generic or brand name of the prescribed medicine. Check to see if the patient has any allergies to the drug that is going to be administered.
4. Right route. Administer the medicine by the prescribed anatomical route and site.
5. Right time, right frequency. Administer the medicine at the prescribed time and frequency.
6. Right dose. Confirm through arithmetical calculation that the dose of the medicine being prescribed concurs exactly with the dose prescribed.
7. Right documentation. Sign, date and retain all documentation recording the administration of each medicine in the medication administration chart or other direction to administer them. The chart must only be signed to record that a medicine has been administered once the medicine administration has been witnessed.
8. Right action. Ensure that the medicine is prescribed for the appropriate reason and state to the patient the action of the medicine, and the reason it has been prescribed.
9. Right form. Confirm that the form of medicine that has been dispensed matches with the specified route of administration.
10. Right response. Observe the patient for adverse effects and assess the patient to determine that the desired effect of the medicines has been achieved.

Medicines can be administered by a single qualified nurse or by two nurses checking – this is known as 'double checking'. Double checking is required when administering controlled drugs (MDA Schedule 2; see below) and when administering drugs via the intravenous route.

If a registered nurse delegates any aspect of the administration of a medicinal product, they are responsible and accountable for ensuring that the patient or health care assistant is competent to carry out the task (NMBI 2015b).

Student nurses must never administer medicines unless they are being directly supervised by a registered nurse. Both the student and the registered nurse must sign the medication chart.

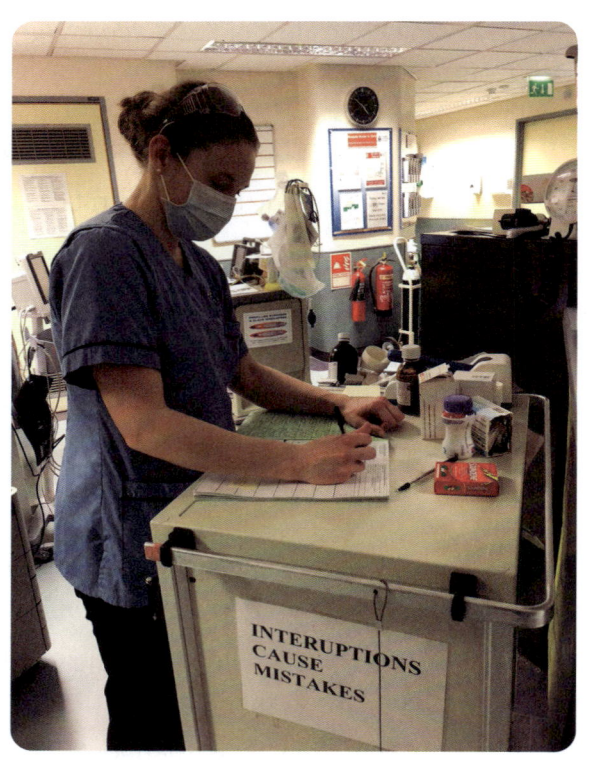

## CONTROLLED DRUGS: MISUSE OF DRUGS ACTS (MDA)

Under the Misuse of Drugs Acts 1977 and 1984, and the MDA Regulations of 1988 (and its amendments), controlled drugs (mainly known for their narcotic or psychotropic characteristics) have been categorised into distinct groups known as schedules.

These schedules, with their additional controls such as record-keeping and storage, are based on the active substances of the drug, their medicinal value and the potential for misuse. Specifically, the Misuse of Drugs Acts direct the level of controls and restrictions for these drugs.

There are five MDA schedules:

* Schedule 1 – drugs that are not used in clinical practice, but in research and forensics, e.g. raw opium.

* Schedule 2 – Schedule 2 drugs are dangerous if misused and thus have greater controls placed on them. Pharmacists may only supply these drugs based on a handwritten prescription. There are strict record-

keeping requirements that nurses must be aware of for managing MDA Schedule 2 drugs. An MDA Schedule 2 controlled drug register must be used. Safe custody and storage must also be maintained. Destruction of these drugs must be witnessed and recorded. Examples include morphine and diamorphine, pethidine and fentanyl.

- Schedule 3 – Less strict controls apply to these drugs. Safe custody provisions and MDA controlled drug prescription writing requirements apply to them. Examples are some analgesics, some stimulants and some benzodiazepines.

- Schedule 4 – While control of these drugs is minimal in practice, they should be supplied in accordance with the Medicinal Products Regulations 2003. It is not required to keep records of these drugs in an MDA controlled drug register or to retain invoices. The regulations for safe custody do not apply. Examples include most benzodiazepines and phenobarbitone.

- Schedule 5 – The drugs listed in this schedule are exempt from the majority of MDA regulations, e.g. codeine and other painkillers.

## MANAGEMENT OF MDA SCHEDULE 2 DRUGS

The local health service provider, whether an acute hospital or a community setting, is obliged to put in place a system whereby the following controls can be implemented by nurses and midwives:

- MDA Schedule 2 drugs should be stored separately from other medicines and at an increased level of safekeeping. They are stored in a locked cupboard within a locked cupboard.

- Double checking by two registered nurses is required when administering these drugs.

- The second person must:
  - check that the prescription is written for the MDA drug
  - check the drug against the prescription
  - add a second signature to the MDA controlled drugs register
  - check the identity of the patient
  - witness the administration of the MDA drug to the patient.

# Recording and documentation

The quality of records maintained by nurses and midwives reflects the quality of the care provided to the patient (NMBI 2015a). Clear and accurate recording of drug administration is necessary to ensure the provision of safe and effective care to the patient. It provides documentary evidence of the care provided and is a legal requirement.

All prescriptions, whether written on an individual prescription sheet or on a medication chart, must be legible and contain the appropriate information about the patient and the prescribed drug.

When administering medication, the nurse must sign and date the medication chart when the medicine administration has been carried out (see Appendix 4 Medication Chart).

# Medication errors

Nurses are accountable for all actions and omissions relating to their role in administering a prescribed medicine. Nurses are accountable for their practice and it is a nurse's own responsibility to keep abreast of changes in practice by engaging in continuing professional development. Nurses can be sanctioned by the regulatory body if an incident occurs due to negligent behaviour. Each individual nurse must only engage in practice that they are competent to do. This level of competence is unique to each nurse and is referred to as his/her 'scope of practice'. We will be discussing this in more detail in the next chapter.

When mistakes do happen, it is the policy of the HSE that healthcare staff communicate to patients in an open, honest, transparent and empathic manner. Following patient safety incidents, staff are required to act promptly, to acknowledge their error and to make an apology where a person is harmed as a result of a medication error or any other type of error. This is referred to as 'open disclosure' and it is the policy adopted by healthcare systems across the world.

# REVISION QUESTIONS

1. In Irish law, which healthcare professionals can prescribe drugs?
2. Which organisation provides guidance to nurses on medication administration?
3. List the seven guiding principles for medication management outlined in the NMBI's *Guidance for Registered Nurses and Midwives on Medication Administration*.
4. In your own words, explain the following terms:
   - Pharmacology
   - Indication for a drug
   - Contraindication for a drug
   - Drug interaction
   - Side effect
   - Polypharmacy
   - Controlled drug
5. Explain why precision and accuracy are important in drug administration.
6. In relation to the following prescription instructions, explain the route and frequency for administration:
   - Augmentin 500 mg PO TDS
   - Normison 20 mg PO nocte
   - Difene Supp 100 mg PR BD
   - Paracetamol 500 mg IV QDS
   - Aspirin 500 mg PO mane
7. List the ten rights that nurses must adhere to for drug administration.
8. When administering a medication, when should the nurse sign and date the drug chart?
9. What should a nurse do if a mistake is made when administering a drug?

# Scope of Practice

In this chapter you will learn about:

* Professional socialisation
* The guidance for determining scope of practice in Ireland
* How an individual nurse determines his/her scope of practice

## Introduction

In Chapter 1 we looked at the development of nursing as a profession. We followed the trajectory of nursing as it evolved from an apprenticeship model to one where nurses achieve a Level 8 honours degree following a four-year course of study that includes clinical instruction.

During clinical practice there is the opportunity for 'professional socialisation'. This is the process where students are exposed to nursing values during the nursing programme as they observe the behaviour of qualified professional nurses.

Student nurses initially observe nurses in practice. As they progress through their undergraduate programme, students participate in practice under the supervision of experienced nurses. By the time a student reaches their nursing internship they have a clear understanding of the role of the nurse. They have learned the values and the norms of nursing. They understand how and why nurses act as they do, what is expected of them and what their responsibilities are. They understand that nurses are accountable for their actions. They understand that the role of the nurse can vary depending on the area of healthcare delivery they are working in. A nurse in an operating theatre is competent in different skills from those of a nurse working in a medical ward. Each of these areas hold different responsibilities.

A nursing qualification provides the holder with a broad range of skills that are adapted according to the area of specialism that the nurse decides to pursue.

> ### Exercise
>
> Imagine you are a nurse working in an intensive care unit. Outline the skills you would need, the activities you would be involved in and what you think your main responsibilities would be.
>
> Repeat this exercise for other nursing roles, e.g. a nurse in a surgical ward, a midwife in a labour ward, a nurse in an accident and emergency department, a nurse manager on a medical ward.
>
> Discuss the similarities and the differences between these nursing roles.

Each nursing role is unique depending on the area of specialism, the service provided, the needs of the patients in that area and the knowledge and experience of the nurse. The term 'scope of practice' refers to the range of roles, functions, responsibilities and activities that a registered nurse or registered midwife is educated, competent and has the authority to perform.

Scope of practice for nurses and midwives in Ireland is determined by legislation, EU directives, international developments, social policy, national and local guidelines, education and individual levels of competence.

The NMBI has developed a framework for nurses and midwives to guide them in determining their roles and responsibilities. It encourages them to critically examine their individual scope of practice in relation to providing safe, high-quality care to patients (NMBI 2015b).

The framework fulfils several functions:

* It underpins decision-making related to nurses' and midwives' everyday practice.
* It helps nurses and midwives to identify professional development needs.
* It provides a basis for the expansion of nursing and midwifery roles.
* It encourages reflective practice to improve learning and the provision of safe, good-quality patient care.

As an enabling framework it also emphasises nurses' and midwives' individual accountability in making decisions about their roles and responsibilities and it is, therefore, an empowering resource for practitioners.

The framework discusses key factors that nurses and midwives need to consider when making decisions about their own scope of practice and outlines the principles that should guide nurses and midwives in reviewing and expanding their scope of practice.

It is the responsibility of each registered nurse and midwife to determine their own scope of practice.

The scope framework builds on the principles, values and standards of conduct of the *Code of Professional Conduct and Ethics* 2014 and introduces new considerations for nurses and midwives in determining their scope of practice.

Nursing and midwifery practice responds to the ever-changing needs of the population and to changes in healthcare delivery. The framework encourages nurses to be proactive in identifying areas where they could expand their scope of practice where it would improve patient outcomes and the quality and the range of services provided. An example of this is the expansion of nurses' scope of practice to include prescribing medications for patients. The legislation for this was passed in 2007 and since then nurses who have undergone additional education programmes have been able to include prescribing in their scope of practice.

We will use an example to demonstrate how this translates into practice. In some acute hospitals, accident and emergency departments have advanced nurse practitioners who provide a nurse-led minor injury service. These nurses were able to examine and assess patients and treat certain injuries; but they could not prescribe medication, e.g. pain relief or antibiotics. When they expanded their scope of practice to include prescribing, they could complete the patient journey without having to call a medical colleague to write the prescription. In order to expand their scope of practice, the nurses had to undergo the nurse prescribing education programme. They had to ensure that they could be accountable for their practice. Their increased knowledge and the development of policies to guide their practice ensured this. They also engaged in continuing professional development to keep themselves up to date with changes in prescribing methods.

# Determining the scope of nursing and midwifery practice

* **Competence.** Competence is the ability to carry out a role or an activity safely. To be competent the nurse must have the necessary knowledge and skill. Levels of competence change over time with increased knowledge and experience. Nurses are encouraged to revise their scope of practice as their competencies change.

* **Responsibility, accountability and autonomy.** This refers to the professional autonomy of nurses and midwives; in other words, their ability to make their own decisions in relation to their practice. Where nurses make those decisions, they are accountable for them. Remember that a nurse must be registered with the NMBI, which holds each nurse accountable and responsible for the actions they take.

* **Continuing professional development.** Nurses are lifelong learners, as are all professionals. Nursing research is carried out continuously and provides the evidence for changes in practice that will improve outcomes for patients. In order to provide effective, good-quality care, nurses must keep themselves abreast of these changes and they do that by engaging in continuing professional development.

* **Support for professional nursing and midwifery practice.** Nursing and midwifery practice is supported by local policies, procedures and guidelines that are based on legislation, regulation and evidence from research.

* **Delegation and supervision.** Nurses and midwives work as members of a multidisciplinary team. Some of the members of that team will be regulated professionals (e.g. other nurses, medics, physiotherapists) and some will be unregulated (e.g. health care assistants). Nurses in the team may delegate tasks to others and when doing so they are accountable for ensuring that the delegated role or activity is appropriate to the level of competence of the person to whom it is delegated. Similarly, where a nurse or a midwife has a particular role or activity delegated to them, they should only undertake it if they are sure that they have the competency to carry it out.

* **Practice setting.** Nurses and midwives may practice in a wide variety of settings, e.g. acute hospital wards, residential care settings, operating theatres, prisons, patients' homes, etc. Nurses and midwives should have the appropriate skill set for the setting.

# Scope of Practice Decision-Making Flowchart

**Think about your Nursing or Midwifery Role or Activity**
**PATIENT SAFETY FIRST**

Is the role/activity you are about to undertake respectful of the patient's rights and will they derive an overall benefit from your actions?

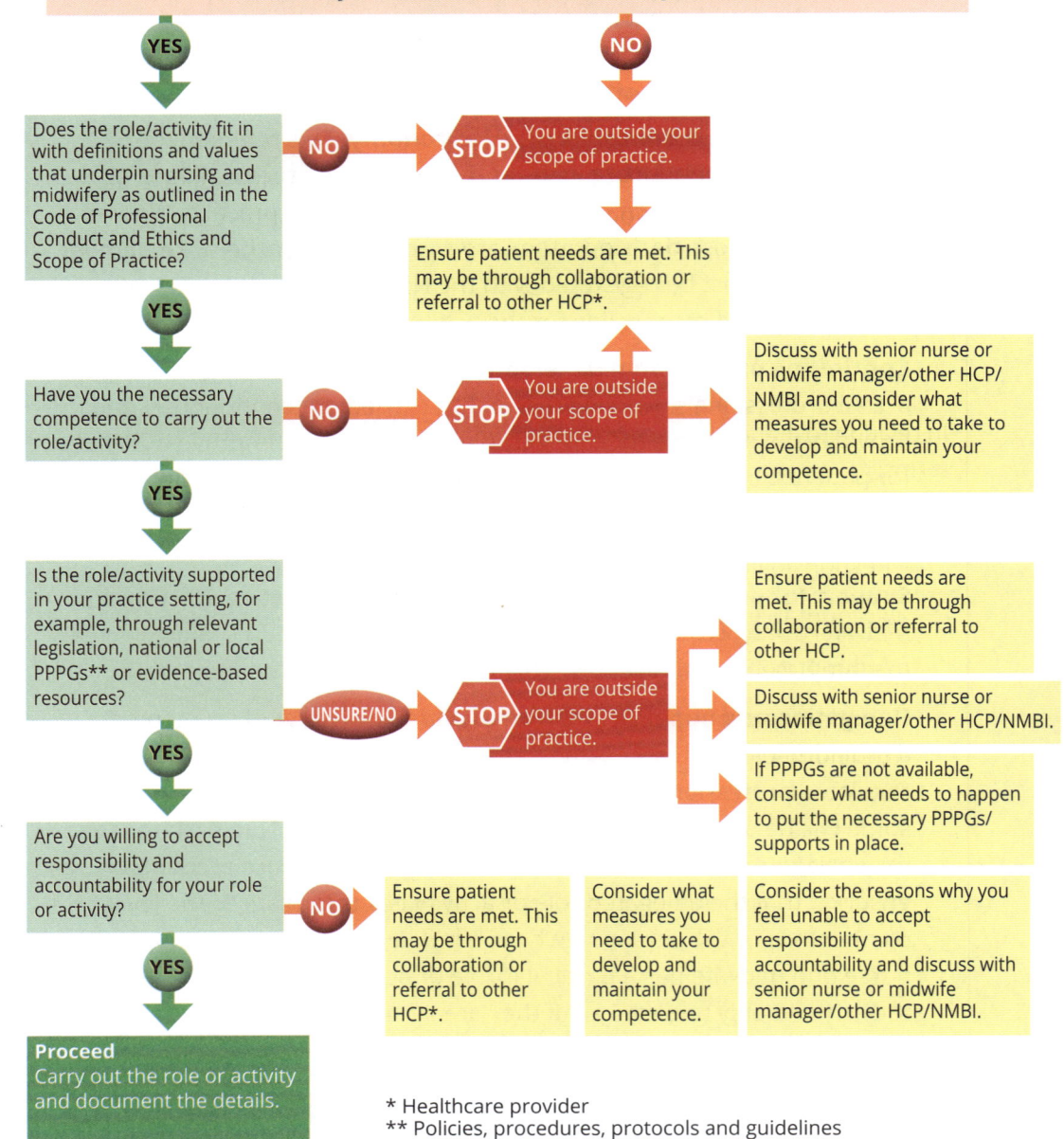

- **YES** ↓
- **NO** → **STOP** You are outside your scope of practice. → Ensure patient needs are met. This may be through collaboration or referral to other HCP*.

**Does the role/activity fit in with definitions and values that underpin nursing and midwifery as outlined in the Code of Professional Conduct and Ethics and Scope of Practice?**
- **NO** → **STOP** You are outside your scope of practice. → Ensure patient needs are met. This may be through collaboration or referral to other HCP*.
- **YES** ↓

**Have you the necessary competence to carry out the role/activity?**
- **NO** → **STOP** You are outside your scope of practice. → Discuss with senior nurse or midwife manager/other HCP/NMBI and consider what measures you need to take to develop and maintain your competence.
- **YES** ↓

**Is the role/activity supported in your practice setting, for example, through relevant legislation, national or local PPPGs** or evidence-based resources?**
- **UNSURE/NO** → **STOP** You are outside your scope of practice. →
  - Ensure patient needs are met. This may be through collaboration or referral to other HCP.
  - Discuss with senior nurse or midwife manager/other HCP/NMBI.
  - If PPPGs are not available, consider what needs to happen to put the necessary PPPGs/supports in place.
- **YES** ↓

**Are you willing to accept responsibility and accountability for your role or activity?**
- **NO** →
  - Ensure patient needs are met. This may be through collaboration or referral to other HCP*.
  - Consider what measures you need to take to develop and maintain your competence.
  - Consider the reasons why you feel unable to accept responsibility and accountability and discuss with senior nurse or midwife manager/other HCP/NMBI.
- **YES** ↓

**Proceed**
Carry out the role or activity and document the details.

\* Healthcare provider
\*\* Policies, procedures, protocols and guidelines

*Source:* NMBI, 2015

* **Collaborative practice.** Where multiple health workers from different professional backgrounds work together with patients, each professional has the responsibility of informing the others about their scope of practice. This requires good communication and respectful relationships between professionals. The goal of collaborative practice is always the provision of safe, effective, good-quality care to patients.

* **Expanded practice.** Where nurses and midwives are competent to include roles or activities that they had not previously undertaken they can expand their scope of practice to do so. Each nurse or midwife is responsible for defining their own scope.

When determining their scope of practice the nurse or midwife will take all these factors into consideration. They will also be guided by the *Code of Professional Conduct and Ethics for Registered Nurses and Midwives* (NMBI 2014).

## REVISION QUESTIONS

In relation to a nurse's practice, explain what you understand by the following terms:

* Competence
* Responsibility
* Accountability
* Autonomy
* Continuing professional development
* Delegation and supervision
* Practice setting
* Collaborative practice
* Expanded practice

# 14

# Commonly Used Terms in Healthcare

In this chapter you will learn about:

* The origins of medical terms
* Abbreviations
* Common medical abbreviations

## Medical terms

Many medical terms originate from Ancient Greece and Rome. They include terms to describe body systems, bodily organs and their functions. An understanding of medical terms helps healthcare professionals to understand each other. A nurse's dictionary is an essential purchase for every student nurse.

Correct spelling is vitally important; the incorrect spelling of a word or term could affect the care of a patient.

There are three components to many medical terms: roots/combining forms; prefixes; and suffixes.

A word **root** is the basic foundation of a word which gives general meaning. Roots are usually combined using a vowel (usually i or o); this is referred to as a combining form. For example:

- Cardi – heart
- Pulmon – lungs
- Haemat – blood
- Gastro – stomach

**Prefixes** are added to the beginning of a word root to change its meaning or create a new word, for example:

- Tachy – fast/rapid, e.g. tachycardia
- Brady – slow, e.g. bradycardia
- Hypo – low, e.g. hypothermia
- Hyper – high, e.g. hyperthermia

**Suffixes** are placed at the end of a word to tell us what is happening to a particular body part, for example:

- -itis – inflammation, e.g. appendicitis, tonsillitis
- -ology – study of, e.g. pathology

# Abbreviations

Full text is always preferable to abbreviations. If you use abbreviations, they should be from an approved list from the healthcare facility or from the HSE's *Code of Practice for Healthcare Records Management* (HSE 2010).

**A**

| | | | |
|---|---|---|---|
| ABC | Airway, breathing, circulation | Anaes. | Anaesthetic |
| Abd. | Abdominal | ANP | Advanced nurse practitioner |
| AD | Alzheimer's disease | Ant. | Anterior |
| ADL | Activities of daily living | APH | Ante partum haemorrhage |
| Adm. | Admission/admitted | | |
| ADON/M | Assistant director of nursing/midwifery | Approx. | Approximately |
| | | Appt. | Appointment |
| AIDS | Acquired immune deficiency syndrome | ASAP | As soon as possible |
| | | Ass. | Assistance |
| a.m. | Morning – before twelve noon | Ausc. | Auscultation |
| | | Ax. | Assessment |

## B

| | | | |
|---|---|---|---|
| Ba. | Barium | BMI | Body mass index |
| BBA | Born before admission/arrival | BMR | Basal metabolic rate |
| | | BNO | Bowels not open |
| BC | Blood cultures | BO | Bowels opened |
| b.d./b.i.d. | Twice daily | BOS | Base of support |
| BG | Blood glucose/blood gases | BP | Blood pressure |
| | | BPM | Beats per minute |
| BGL | Blood glucose level | Bx. | Biopsy |

## C

| | | | |
|---|---|---|---|
| Ca. | Carcinoma | Cons. | Consultant |
| CAD | Coronary artery disease | Cont'd. | Continued |
| cc | Copied to | COPD | Chronic obstructive pulmonary disease |
| CCF | Congestive cardiac failure | | |
| CCU | Coronary care unit | CRF | Chronic renal failure |
| Chemo | Chemotherapy | CandS | Culture and sensitivity |
| CHO | Carbohydrate | CS | Caesarean section |
| Chol. | Cholesterol | CSE | Combined spinal epidural |
| CLD | Chronic lung disease | CSF | Cerebrospinal fluid |
| cm | Centimetre | CSU | Catheter specimen of urine |
| CMM 1, 2, 3 | Clinical midwife manager 1, 2, 3 | CT | Computerised tomography |
| CNM 1, 2, 3 | Clinical nurse manager 1, 2, 3 | CV | Cardiovascular |
| CNS | Central nervous system | CVA | Cerebrovascular accident |
| $CO_2$ | Carbon dioxide | CVL | Central venous line |
| CO | Complaining of | CVP | Central venous pressure |
| COLD | Chronic obstructive lung disease | CVS | Cardiovascular system |
| | | Cx. | Cervix |
| Conc. | Concentration | CxR | Chest X-ray |

## D

| | | | |
|---|---|---|---|
| DBE | Deep breathing exercises | DOM/N | Director of midwifery/nursing |
| DandC | Dilatation and curettage | DPM | Drops per minute |
| Dc. | Discharge | Dr. | Doctor |
| Defib. | Defibrillation | DTs | Delirium tremens |
| Dept. | Department | DandV | Diarrhoea and vomiting |
| DM | Diabetes mellitus | DVT | Deep vein thrombosis |
| DNA | Did not attend | DW | Discussed with |
| DOA | Dead on arrival | Dx/Δ | Diagnosis |
| DOB | Date of birth | | |

## E

| | | | |
|---|---|---|---|
| EA | Elective admission | EDD | Estimated date of delivery |
| EBL | Estimated blood loss | e.g. | For example |
| ECG | Electrocardiogram | Enc. | Enclosed |
| ECHO | Echocardiogram | ENT | Ear, nose and throat |
| E. Coli | Escherichia coli | Est. Req. | Estimated requirements |
| ECT | Electroconvulsive therapy | EUA | Examination under anaesthetic |
| ED | Emergency department | | |

## F

| | | | |
|---|---|---|---|
| FB | Foreign body | FHHR | Foetal heart heard and regular |
| FBC | Full blood count | FMF | Foetal movement felt |
| FBS | Fasting blood sugar | FOB | Faecal occult blood |
| Fe | Iron | FU | Follow up |
| FFP | Fresh frozen plasma | FWB | Full weight bearing |
| FH | Foetal heart | | |

## G

| | | | |
|---|---|---|---|
| g | Gram | GIT | Gastro-intestinal tract |
| GA | General anaesthetic | GO | Gastro-oesophageal |
| GBS | Group B Streptococcus | GORD | Gastro-oesophageal reflux disorder/disease |
| GCS | Glasgow coma scale | GP | General practitioner |
| gest. | Gestation | GTT | Glucose tolerance test |
| GF | Gluten-free | GU | Genito-urinary |
| G&H | Group and hold | GXM | Group and cross match |
| GI | Gastro-intestinal | | |

## H

| | | | |
|---|---|---|---|
| H | Hour | HIV | Human immunodeficiency virus |
| Haem. | Haematology | HR | Heart rate |
| Hams. | Hamstrings | HRT | Hormone replacement therapy |
| Hb | Haemoglobin | | |
| HC | Head circumference | HSE | Health Service Executive |
| HCA | Home care assistant | Ht. | Height |
| HDU | High dependency unit | HTN | Hypertension |
| Hep. A/B/C | Hepatitis A/B/C | HV | Home visit |
| HH | Home help | HVS | High vaginal swab |
| HI | Head injury | Hx. | History |

## I

| | | | |
|---|---|---|---|
| ICU | Intensive care unit | In Pt. | In-patient |
| I&D | Incision and drainage | INR | International normalised ratio |
| ID | Infectious disease | | |
| i.e. | that is | ITT | Insulin tolerance test |
| Ig | Immunoglobulin | ITU | Intensive therapy unit |
| IHD | Ischaemic heart disease | IU | International unit |
| IHF | Irish Heart Foundation | IUD | Intrauterine contraceptive device |
| IM | Intramuscular | | |
| Imp. | Impression | IV | Intravenous |
| Incl. | Including/included | IVI | Intravenous infusion |
| Ind. | Independent | IWA | Irish Wheelchair Association |
| Inf. | Inferior | | |
| Info. | Information | Ix. | Investigation |

## K

| | | | |
|---|---|---|---|
| k+ | Potassium | kg. | kilogram |
| kcal | Kilocalorie | kJ | kilojoules |
| kCL | Potassium chloride | | |

## L

| | | | |
|---|---|---|---|
| L | Litre | LOC | Loss of consciousness |
| LA | Local anaesthetic | LP | Lumbar puncture |
| Lab. | Laboratory | LSCS | Lower segment caesarean section |
| Lat. | Lateral | | |
| lbs. | Pounds weight | LTC | Long-term care |
| LFTs | Liver function tests | LTM | Long-term memory |
| LIF | Left iliac fossa | LVF | Left ventricular failure |
| LIH | Left inguinal hernia | Ly. | Lying |

## M

| | | | |
|---|---|---|---|
| Mane | Morning | mmol | millimole |
| MAU | Medical assessment/admission unit | MMR | Measles, mumps, rubella |
| | | MND | Motor neurone disease |
| Max. | Maximum | Mob. | Mobility/mobilising |
| MDT | Multidisciplinary team | MRI | Magnetic resonance imaging |
| Meds. | Medication | | |
| Mets. | Metastases | MROP | Manual removal of placenta |
| mg | Milligram | | |
| $Mg^{2+}$ | Magnesium | MRSA | Methicillin-resistant *Staphylococcus aureus* |
| MI | Myocardial infarction | | |
| Micro. | Microbiology | MS | Multiple sclerosis |
| Min. | Minimum | Msg. | Message |
| Mins. | Minutes | MSSA | Methicillin-sensitive *Staphylococcus aureus* |
| mL | Millilitre | | |
| mm | Millimetre | MSU | Midstream specimen of urine |
| mmHg | millimetres of mercury | | |

## N

| | | | |
|---|---|---|---|
| $N_2O$ | Nitrous oxide | NFA | No fixed abode |
| NA | Not applicable | NFR | Not for resuscitation |
| $Na^+$ | Sodium | Ng | Naso-gastric |
| NaCL | Sodium chloride | NH | Nursing home |
| NAD | No abnormality detected | NKA | No known allergies |
| NB | Important | NkDA | No known drug allergies |
| Neg. | Negative | No. | Number |
| Neuro. | Neurological | Nocte | Night |

| NOF | Neck of femur | NSAID | Non-steroidal anti-inflammatory drug(s) |
| NOK | Next of kin | | |
| NP | New patient | N&V | Nausea and vomiting |
| NPO | Nil per oral | NWB | Non-weight bearing |
| NPU | Not passed urine | | |

## O

| $O_2$ | Oxygen | OE | On examination |
| OA | Osteoarthritis | Onc. | Oncology |
| OAusc. | On auscultation | OP | Outpatient |
| Obj. | Objective | OPD | Outpatient department |
| Obs. | Observations | Ortho. | Orthopaedics |
| Occ. | Occasional | OT | Occupational therapy/therapist |
| OD | Overdose | | |

## P

| Paeds. | Paediatrics | POP | Plaster of Paris |
| PCA | Patient-controlled analgesia | Pos. | Positive |
| | | Post. | Posterior |
| PE | Pulmonary embolus/embolism | Post Op. | Post operation |
| | | PR | Per rectum |
| PEARL | Pupils equal and reacting to light | Prem. | Premature |
| | | Premed. | Premedication |
| PHN | Public health nurse | | |
| Physio. | Physiotherapist/physiotherapy | Pre Op | Pre-operation |
| | | p.r.n. | Pro re nata (as required) |
| PID | Pelvic inflammatory disease | PTSD | Post-traumatic stress disorder |
| PKU | Phenylketonuria | | |
| PLTS | Platelets | PU | Passed urine |
| p.m. | Afternoon | PUD | Peptic ulcer disease |
| PMHx. | Past medical history | PV | Per vagina |
| PO | Per oral (by mouth) | | |

## Q

| q.d.s./q.i.d. | Four times daily | Quads. | Quadriceps |

## R

| | | | |
|---|---|---|---|
| RBC | Red blood cells | Rh. | Rhesus |
| RBg | Random blood glucose | RICE | Rest, ice, compression, elevation |
| RC | Roman Catholic | | |
| RCN | Registered children's nurse | RIF | Right iliac fossa |
| | | RIP | Rest in peace/deceased |
| RD | Retinal detachment | RLQ | Right lower quadrant |
| RDS | Respiratory distress syndrome | RM | Registered midwife |
| | | RO | Removal of |
| Re. | Regarding | RR | Respiratory/respiration rate |
| Rec'd | Received | | |
| Recom. | Recommended | RT | Radiotherapy |
| Reg. | Registrar | RTA | Road traffic accident |
| Rehab. | Rehabilitation | RTI | Respiratory tract infection |
| REM | Rapid eye movement | | |
| Reps. | Repetition | Rv. | Review |
| Resp. | Respiration | RV | Right ventricle |
| Rev. | Revision | Rx. | Treatment |
| RgN | Registered general nurse | | |

## S

| | | | |
|---|---|---|---|
| s | Second (time) | SLT | Speech and language therapy/therapist |
| SA | Spinal anaesthetic | | |
| SAD | Seasonal affective disorder | Snr. | Senior |
| | | SOB | Shortness of breath |
| SAH | Sub arachnoid haemorrhage | SR | Sinus rhythm |
| | | ST | Sinus tachycardia |
| $SaO_2$ | Oxygen saturation | STAT | At once/immediately |
| SB | Seen by | Stats. | Statistics |
| SBR | Serum bilirubin rate | STM | Short-term memory |
| SC | Subcutaneous | Surg. | Surgical |
| SIDS | Sudden infant death syndrome | | |

## T

| | | | |
|---|---|---|---|
| TB | Tuberculosis | TF | Transfer |
| TBL | Total blood loss | TIA | Transient ischaemic attack |
| TCI | To come in | | |
| T1DM | Type 1 diabetes mellitus | TPN | Total parenteral nutrition |
| T2DM | Type 2 diabetes mellitus | TPR | Temperature, pulse and respiration |
| t.d.s./t.i.d. | Three times daily | | |
| TEDS | Thrombo-embolic deterrent stockings | Ts and As | Tonsillectomy and adenoidectomy |
| Temp. | Temperature | TSH | Thyroid stimulating hormone |

## U

| | | | |
|---|---|---|---|
| UA | Urinalysis | US/USS | Ultrasound/ultrasound scan |
| UC | Urinary catheter | | |
| U&E | Urea and electrolytes | UST | Ultrasound therapy |
| UO | Urinary output | UTI | Urinary tract infection |
| URTI | Upper respiratory tract infection | | |

## V

| | | | |
|---|---|---|---|
| Via | By way of | VVs | Varicose veins |
| Vol. | Volume | Vx. | Vertex |
| VT | Ventricular tachycardia | | |

## W

| | | | |
|---|---|---|---|
| WB | Weight bear/bearing | W.end | Weekend |
| WBC | Whole blood count | WL | Waiting list |
| WC | Water closet/toilet | WNL | Within normal limits |
| WCC | White cell count | WR | Ward round |
| W.chair | Wheelchair | Wt. | Weight |

## X

| | |
|---|---|
| x-match | Crossmatch |

## Y

| | |
|---|---|
| YO | Year old |

## Z

| | |
|---|---|
| Zn | Zinc |

| | |
|---|---|
| & | And |
| @ | At |
| # | Fracture |
| ? | Query |
| x2 | Twice |
| ° | Degrees – only permitted for measuring angles Δ |
| °C | Temperature in degrees Celsius |

# Glossary

**Accountability** – being answerable for one's judgments, actions, and omissions as they relate to professional nursing practice

**Advocacy** – a means of empowering people by supporting them to assert their views and claim their entitlements, and, where necessary, representing and negotiating on their behalf

**Anatomy** – the study of the normal structure of the human body

**Autonomy** – a person's ability to make choices on the basis of her or his preferences, beliefs and values

**Axilla** – area in the armpit

**Blood-borne virus** – a virus that is carried in the blood

**Chain of infection** – a graphical description of how cross-infection occurs

**Colonisation** – when pathogens are present on the body but have not invaded the body to cause infection

**Community care** – the provision of care in the person's own home or within their community

**Competence** – the ability to put knowledge and theory into practice in a safe and effective manner

**Conduct** – a person's moral practices, actions, beliefs and standards of behaviour

**Confidential** – something that is private or secret

**Consent** – to give one's permission

**Cross-infection** – when a micro-organism passes from one person to another

**Dignity** – having respect for someone's worth

**Empathy** – the ability to imagine the experience of another person

**Ethics –** the principles, values and virtues that enable people to live a morally good life

**Evidence-based practice –** nursing practice that is based on scientific research and sound knowledge

**Healthcare-associated infection –** an infection that is acquired after contact with health services

**Holistic care –** care that is provided based on an assessment of the person's entire needs

**Homeostasis –** the body's natural inclination to achieve balance and maintain equilibrium

**Independence –** being self-reliant and able to function on one's own

**In situ –** when something stays in the same place for a period of time

**Intravenous –** in the vein

**Mandatory –** a legal requirement to take an action

**Manual handling –** transporting or supporting a load, moving it from one place to another

**Microbiology –** the study of micro-organisms

**Micro-organisms –** tiny living cells that can only be seen through a microscope

**Mode of transmission –** the different methods by which pathogens can spread from one person to another

**Multidisciplinary team –** a healthcare team consisting of members of different healthcare professions

**Pathogen –** a disease-causing micro-organism

**People moving and handling –** assisting people that have difficulty with mobility

**Person –** an individual who uses health and social care services

**Person centred care –** an approach to care that places the person at the centre of the design and delivery of care

**Predisposing factor –** a factor that increases the likelihood of something occurring

**Primary care –** care that is provided at the first point of contact with health services

**Reflective practice –** a conscious review of an event, situation, information or emotion encountered with the aim of analyzing and evaluating the experience to apply insights to future practice

**Regulation –** something that is compulsory and a necessary condition for achievement or approval

**Respect –** having due regard for a person's feelings, wishes and/or rights to receive appropriate care

**Responsibility –** the obligation to perform duties, tasks or roles based on sound professional judgment

**Scope of practice –** the range of roles, functions, responsibilities and activities which a registered nurse is educated, competent and has authority to perform

**Secondary care –** care that is provided in acute hospitals

**Sepsis –** a systemic inflammatory response that can progress to cause organ failure and ultimately death

**Standard precautions –** a range of practices that healthcare workers can apply in their work setting, designed to reduce the risk of cross-infection

**Sympathy –** having pity or sorrow for another person

**Tertiary care –** highly specialised care

**Therapeutic relationship –** the relationship established and maintained between a person requiring or receiving care and a nurse

**Transmission-based precautions –** additional precautions implemented when a person has a known infection or is suspected of having an infection

**Voluntary –** done of free will

# References

Alfaro-LeFevre, R. (2014) *Applying Nursing Process: The Foundation for Clinical Reasoning* (8th edn). Philadelphia: Wolters Kluwer/Lippincott Williams & Wilkins.

Bach, S. and Grant, A. (2010) *Communication and Interpersonal Skills in Nursing*. London: Learning Matters.

Baxter, R., Ray, G.T. and Fireman, B.H. (2008) 'Case-control Study of Antibiotic Use and Subsequent Clostridium Difficile Associated Diarrhoea in Hospitalized Patients.' Infection Control & Hospital Epidemiology. January 29(1):44–50.

Benner, P., Tanner, C.A. and Chesla, C.A. (1996) *Expertise in Nursing Practice: Caring, Clinical Judgment, and Ethics* (2nd edn). New York: Springer.

Bostridge. M. (2008) *Florence Nightingale: The Woman and Her Legend*. London: Penguin Viking.

Chowdhry, S. (2010) 'Exploring the concept of empathy in nursing: can it lead to abuse of patient trust?', *Nursing Times* 106(42).

Commission on Nursing (1998) *Report of the Commission on Nursing: A Blueprint for the Future*. Dublin: Stationery Office.

Condell, I., Faherty, S. and Fitzpatrick, M. (2014) 'Knowledge and experiences of newly qualified prescribers in Ireland', *Nurse Prescribing* 12(10).

Docherty, C. and McCallum, J. (2009) *Foundation Clinical Nursing Skills*. Oxford: Oxford University Press.

DoH (Department of Health) (1980) *Working Party on General Nursing Report*. Dublin: Stationery Office.

— (2016) *Values for Nurses and Midwives* (Position Paper 1) <https://www.nmbi.ie/NMBI/media/NMBI/Position-Paper-Values-for-Nurses-and-Midwives-June-2016.pdf>. Dublin: Department of Health.

— (2020). Irish National Early Warning System V2 (NCEC National Clinical Guideline No. 1). <https://www.gov.ie/en/collection/c9fa9a-national-clinical-guidelines/>.

DoHC (Department of Health and Children) (2001) *Primary Care: A New Direction*. Dublin: Government of Ireland.

Dooley, D. and McCarthy, J. (2012) *Nursing Ethics: Irish Cases and Concerns*. Dublin: Gill Education.

Dougherty, L., Lister, S. and West-Oram, A. (eds) (2015) *The Royal Marsden Manual of Clinical Nursing Procedures* (9th edn). London: Wiley-Blackwell.

EEC (European Economic Community) (1977) Council Directive 77/452/EEC (Recognition of nurses' qualifications).

— (1989) Council Directive 89/595/EEC (Recognition of nurses' qualifications).

Elliott, M. and Liu, Y. (2010) 'The nine rights of medication administration: an overview', *British Journal of Nursing* 19(5): 300–5.

European Union (EU) (2013). Directive 2013/55/EU (Recognition of professional qualifications).

Ewen, J. and Kirkpatrick, P. (2009) 'Personal and Oral Hygiene' in H. Iggulden, C. MacDonald and K. Staniland (eds) *Clinical Skills: The Essence of Caring*. London: Open University Press.

Gibbs, G. (1988) *Learning by Doing: A Guide to Teaching and Learning Methods*. Oxford: Oxford Polytechnic Further Education Unit.

Government of Ireland (1919) The Nurses Registration Act 1919. Dublin: Stationery Office.

— (1950) Nurses Act 1950. Dublin: Stationery Office.

— (1977) Misuse of Drugs Act 1977. Dublin: Stationery Office.

— (1984) Misuse of Drugs Act 1984. Dublin: Stationery Office.

— (1995) Irish Medicines Board Act 1995. Dublin: Stationery Office.

— (2006) Irish Medicines Board (Miscellaneous Provisions) Act 2006. Dublin: Stationery Office.

— (2007a) Pharmacy Act 2007. Dublin: Stationery Office.

— (2007b) Misuse of Drugs (Amendment) Regulations 2007. Statutory Instrument No. 200 of 2007. Dublin: Stationery Office.

— (2014) Misuse of Drugs (Amendment) Regulations 2014. Statutory Instrument No. 323 of 2014. Dublin: Stationery Office.

— (2015) *Strategy for the Office of the Chief Nursing Officer, 2015–2017*. Dublin: Stationery Office.

Grant, A. and Waugh, A. (2018) *Ross and Wilson Anatomy and Physiology on Health and Illness* (13th edn). London: Churchill Livingstone Elsevier.

Health Protection Surveillance Centre (HPSC) (2018) Infectious Disease Notification in Ireland, 2012–2017.

Henderson, V. (1966) *The Basic Principles of Nursing*. Geneva: International Council of Nurses.

HIQA (Health Information and Quality Authority) (2012) *National Standards for Safer Better Healthcare*.

— (2013a) *National Quality Standards for Residential Care Settings for Older People in Ireland*. Dublin: HIQA.

— (2013b) *National Quality Standards for Residential Care Services for Children and Adults with Disabilities in Ireland*. Dublin: HIQA.

— (2014) *Guidance for Health and Social Care Providers: Principles of Good Practice in Medication Reconciliation*. Dublin: HIQA.

— (2015) *Medicines Management Guidance*. Dublin: HIQA.

Holland, K., Jenkins, J., Solomon, J. and Whittam, S. (2003) *Applying the Roper-Logan-Tierney Model in Practice*. London: Churchill Livingstone.

HSA (Health and Safety Authority) (2007) *Guide to the Safety, Health and Welfare at Work (General Applications) Regulations 2007*. Dublin: HSA.

— (2015) *Summary of Workplace Injury, Illness and Fatality Statistics 2014–2015*. Dublin: HSA.

— (2020) *Annual Review of Workplace Injury, Illness and Fatality Statistics 2018–2019*. Dublin: HSA.

HSE (Health Service Executive) (2008) *Strategy for Managing Work-Related Aggression and Violence in the Irish Health Service*. Dublin: HSE.

— (2009) *Standard Precautions* < https://www.hse.ie/eng/about/who/healthwellbeing/infectcont/sth/gl/section-3-full-doc.pdf>.

— (2010) *Code of Practice for Healthcare Records Management* <https://www.hse.ie/eng/about/who/qualityandpatientsafety/safepatientcare/healthrecordsmgt/healthcare-records-management.html>.

— (2012) *Guidelines on Infection Prevention and Control 2012* <https://www.hse.ie/eng/about/who/healthwellbeing/infectcont/sth/gl/ipcc-guidelines-section-20.pdf>.

— (2015a) *Building a High Quality Health Service for a Healthier Ireland. Health Service Executive Corporate Plan 2015–2017* <https://www.hse.ie/eng/services/publications/corporate/corporateplan15-17.pdf>.

— (2015b) *Guidelines for Hand Hygiene in Irish Healthcare Settings: Update of 2005 Guidelines*. HCAI, RCPI, HSE.

— (2016) *Person-Centred Principles and Person-Centred Practice Framework* <https://www.hse.ie/eng/staff/resources/changeguide/resources/person-centred-principles-and-person-centred-practice-framework.pdf>.

— (2017) Standard Precautions <https://www.hse.ie/eng/about/who/healthwellbeing/infectcont/sth/gl/section-3-introduction.pdf>.

HSE and HPSC (2015) Health Service Executive and Health Protection Surveillance Centre (2015) *Annual Epidemiological Report 2014* <https://www.hpsc.ie/aboutpsc/annualreports/annualepidemiologicalreports1999-2016/HPSC%20Annual%20Report%202014%20%20.pdf>.

Hutson, M. and Millar, E. (2009) 'Record Keeping', in H. Iggulden, C. MacDonald and K. Staniland (eds) *Clinical Skills: The Essence of Caring*. London: Open University Press.

ICN (International Council for Nurses) (2012) *ICN Code of Ethics for Nurses*. Geneva: ICN.

Iggulden, H., MacDonald, C. and Staniland, K. (2009) *Clinical Skills: The Essence of Caring*. London: Open University Press.

Ingram, P. and Lavery, I. (2009) *Clinical Skills for Healthcare Assistants*. London: Wiley-Blackwell.

Jamieson, E., McCall, J. and Whyte, L. (2002) *Clinical Nursing Practices*. London: Churchill Livingstone.

Kara, M. (2007) 'Using the Roper, Logan and Tierney Model in care of people with COPD', *Journal of Clinical Nursing* 16(7B): 223–33. DOI: 10.1111/j.1365-2702.2006.01561.x.

LHP Skillnet (2011) *Concepts of Care. A Text Book for Health Care Assistants*. Dublin: LHP Skillnet.

Loughrey, M. (2019) *A Century of Service: A History of the Irish Nurses and Midwives Organisation, 1919–2019*. Dublin: Irish Academic Press.

Moonie, N. (2007) *Advanced Health and Social Care*. Oxford: Heineman.

Neuman, B. (2011) *The Neuman Systems Model* (5th edn; first published 1982). Pearson.

Nightingale, Florence (1992) *Notes on Nursing*, ed. Victor Skretkowicz (first published 1859). Turkey: Scutari Press.

NMBI (Nursing and Midwifery Board of Ireland) (2014) *Code of Professional Conduct and Ethics for Registered Nurses and Midwives* < https://www.nmbi.ie/Standards-Guidance/Code>. Dublin: NMBI.

— (2015a) *Recording Clinical Practice – Professional Guidelines*. Dublin: NMBI.

— (2015b) *Scope of Nursing and Midwifery Practice*. Dublin: NMBI.

— (2016) *Nurse Registration Programmes Standards and Requirements* (4th edn). Dublin: NMBI.

— (2017) *A Guide to Fitness to Practice*. Dublin: NMBI.

— (2019) *Practice Standards for Nurses and Midwives with Prescriptive Authority*. Dublin: NMBI.

— (2020) *Guidance for Registered Nurses and Midwives on Medication Administration*. Dublin: NMBI.

— (2021) *Pre-Registration Honours Degree Programmes 2012: Nursing/Midwifery – A Career for You*. Dublin: NMBI.

Nolan, E. (2013) *Caring for the Nation: A History of the Mater Misericordiae University Hospital*. Dublin: Gill & Macmillan.

Nolan, P. (2005) 'Caring, Past and Present' in G.M. Fealy, *Care to Remember: Nursing and Midwifery in Ireland*. Cork: Mercier Press.

Orem, D. (2001) *Nursing: Concepts of Practice* (6th edn). St Louis, MO: Mosby.

O'Shea, Y. (2008) *Nursing and Midwifery in Ireland: A Strategy for Professional Development in a Changing Health Service*. Dublin: Blackhall.

— (2013) *The Professional Development of Nursing and Midwifery in Ireland: Key Challenges for the Twenty-First Century*. Dublin: Orpen Press.

Power, M. (2008) 'Care Skills', in I. Duffy (ed.), *Healthcare Support: A Textbook for Healthcare Assistants*. Dublin: Gill & Macmillan, pp. 32–49.

Robins, J. (2000) *Nursing and Midwifery in Ireland in the Twentieth Century*. Dublin: An Bord Altranais.

Roper, N., Logan, W.W. and Tierney, A.J. (1980) *The Elements of Nursing*. Edinburgh: Churchill Livingstone.

Schon, D.A. (1991) *The Reflective Turn: Case Studies In and On Educational Practice*. New York: Teachers College Press, Columbia University.

TILDA (Irish Longitudinal Study on Ageing) (2012) *Polypharmacy in Adults over 50 in Ireland: Opportunities for Cost Saving and Improved Healthcare*. Dublin: TILDA.

Tortora, G.J. and Derrickson, B.H. (2014) *Principles of Anatomy and Physiology* (14th edn). Hoboken, N.J.: Wiley.

UCD School of Nursing, Midwifery and Health Systems (n.d.) *Enhancing Person-Centred Care*. <https://www.hse.ie/eng/about/who/qid/leadershipquality/enhancing-person-centred-care-presentation.pdf>.

Van Dokkum, N. (2011) *Nursing Law For Students in Ireland*. Dublin: Gill & Macmillan.

WHO (World Health Organization) (2006) Five Moments for Hand Hygiene <https://www.who.int/gpsc/tools/Five_moments/en/>.

Wright, B. (2007) *Interpersonal Skills*. Keswick, Cumbria: M&K Update.

# Appendices

## Appendix 1 Roper, Logan and Tierney Assessment Sheet

| Patient's Name: _____ | Hospital Number: _____ |
|---|---|
| **ASSESSMENT OF ACTIVITIES OF LIVING** ||
| **Activity of Living** | **Assess Alteration from Patient's Usual Routine and What They Can do or Cannot Do Independently (Please tick)** |
| 1. **Maintaining a Safe Environment**<br>• Change in environment<br>• Change in routine<br>• Change in condition/ impairment<br>• Dependence in maintaining a safe environment<br>• Risks of falls | Identification Bracelet Applied: YES ☐ NO ☐<br>(*Name, Date of Birth, Hospital Number/Address*)<br>Patient orientated to ward: YES ☐ NO ☐<br>Patient confused: NO ☐ YES ☐ (commence care plan)<br>Patient Falls Risk assessment completed: NO ☐ YES ☐ (commence care plan)<br>Intravenous Cannula in situ: NO ☐ YES ☐ (commence care plan) |
| 2. **Communication**<br>• Change in environment<br>• Impaired mode of communication<br>• Dependence in communicating<br>• Discomfort associated with communication | **LANGUAGE/SPEECH:**<br>Patient is able to communicate verbally: YES ☐ NO ☐ (commence care plan) |
| | **HEARING:** Normal ☐ Impaired Hearing ☐ Deaf ☐ (commence care plan)<br>Hearing Aid: YES ☐ NO ☐<br>Hearing Aid is with patient: YES ☐ NO ☐<br>Right Ear ☐ Left Ear ☐ Both Ears ☐ Not Applicable ☐ |
| | **VISION:** Normal ☐ Visually Impaired ☐ Blind ☐<br>(Commence care plan if patient is visually impaired or is blind)<br>Patient wears glasses ☐ Patient wears contact lenses ☐<br>Visual Aid is with patient: YES ☐ NO ☐<br>Please state visual aid: _____<br>Patient has eye prosthesis: YES ☐ NO ☐ |
| | **PAIN ON ADMISSION:** NO ☐ YES ☐ (commence care plan)<br>0 = No Pain  10 = Severe Pain    Pain Score _____<br>Site of pain: _____<br>_____<br>_____<br>_____ |

| | | |
|---|---|---|
| 3. **Breathing**<br>• Respiratory pattern<br>• Difficulty in breathing<br>• Discomfort in breathing | **BREATHING PATTERN:**<br>No breathing difficulties ☐   Breathing difficulties ☐   (commence care plan)<br>Patient is on home oxygen:   YES ☐   NO ☐<br>Patient is on home nebuliser:   YES ☐   NO ☐<br>Patient has a tracheostomy:   YES ☐   NO ☐<br>Patient is a smoker:   YES ☐   NO ☐<br>Number of cigarettes smoked daily: _____ | |
| 4. **Eating and Drinking**<br>• Change in environment/routine<br>• Dependence in eating and drinking<br>• Change in habits<br>• Change in mode (NG, PEG, etc)<br>• Discomfort associated with eating and drinking | Weight: _____ kgs   Height: _____ cms   BMI: _____ kg/m²<br>**APPETITE:** Normal ☐   Increased ☐   Decreased ☐<br>Special diet: _____<br>Assistance required with eating:   None ☐   Partial ☐   Complete ☐<br>Food intake chart commenced:   YES ☐   NO ☐<br>Nausea/Vomiting:   YES ☐   NO ☐<br>Dentures:   YES ☐   NO ☐     Dentures with patient: YES ☐   NO ☐<br>                                                        (on admission)<br>Crowns/Caps/Loose teeth:   YES ☐   NO ☐<br>Difficulty with eating and drinking:   YES ☐   NO ☐<br>Difficulty with swallowing:   YES ☐   NO ☐<br>Difficulty with chewing:   YES ☐   NO ☐<br>Has the patient unplanned weight loss in the page 3–6 months: YES ☐   NO ☐<br>Is there likely to be no nutritional intake for >5 days:   YES ☐   NO ☐<br>Alcohol intake: _____<br>MUST from completed:   YES ☐   NO ☐ | |
| 5. **Eliminating**<br>• Dependence in eliminating<br>• Changes in elimination habits<br>• Change in mode (Catheter, Colostomy etc.)<br>• Discomfort<br>• Loss of control | **MICTURITION:** Altered:   NO ☐   YES ☐   (commence care plan)<br>Describe alteration: _____<br>Urinary Catheter in situ:   NO ☐   YES ☐   Date inserted: _____<br>Catheter Type: _____ Catheter Size: _____<br>**BOWEL PATTERN:** Altered:   NO ☐   YES ☐   (commence care plan)<br>                           Diarrhoea ☐   Constipation ☐<br>Describe any additional alteration:<br>_____<br>Patient uses laxatives:   NO ☐   YES ☐ | |
| 6. **Personal Cleaning and Dressing** | **PERSONAL CARE AND DRESSING:**<br>Self caring ☐   Assistance required ☐   Complete care required ☐<br>Oral cavity assessed:   YES ☐   NO ☐<br>Comment regarding condition of mouth: _____<br>Patient required continued oral hygiene:   YES ☐   NO ☐   (commence care plan)<br>Comment regarding condition of hair: _____ | |
| 7. **Mobilising**<br>• Environment/discomfort<br>• Changes in mobilising habits<br>• Dependence | **MOBILISING:**<br>Independent ☐   Dependent ☐   Requires assistance ☐   (commence care plan)<br>Patient uses mobility aids:   YES ☐   NO ☐<br>Type of Aid used: _____<br>Patient brought in his/her own mobility aid:   YES ☐   NO ☐ | |

| | | |
|---|---|---|
| 8. **Expressing Sexuality**<br>• Difficulty associated with expressive issues, physical disability, disease, disfigurement<br>• Discomfort | Alteration in body image: _____ | |
| | The alteration in body image is due to injury: | YES ☐  NO ☐ |
| | The alteration in body image is due to surgery: | YES ☐  NO ☐ |
| | The alteration in body image is due to medication: | YES ☐  NO ☐ |
| | The alteration in body image is due to instrumentation: | YES ☐  NO ☐ |
| | All the above not applicable: ☐ | |
| 9. **Sleeping**<br>• Change of environment/routine<br>• Sleep disturbances (insomnia, discomforts)<br>• Impaired consciousness Anaesthesia, coma convulsions | Patient currently takes night sedation:       YES ☐  NO ☐<br>Sleeping pattern: _____<br>Alteration in normal sleep pattern:        YES ☐  NO ☐ | |
| 10. **Controlling body temperature** | Apyrexial ☐        Pyrexial ☐        Hypothermic ☐<br>_____<br>_____<br>_____ | |
| 11. **Dying**<br>• Physical problems<br>• Psychological problem<br>• Problems associated with bereavement | Has the patient worries/fears with regard to admission: | YES ☐  NO ☐ |
| | Has the patient worries/fears with regard to tests and investigations: | YES ☐  NO ☐ |
| | Palliative Care referral:        YES ☐ | NO ☐ |
| | Patient requested Priest/Minister:        YES ☐ | NO ☐ |
| 12. **Working/Playing**<br>• Change of environment<br>• Dependence on working/playing<br>• Changes in work/play habits | Patient is concerned about lifestyle changes: | YES ☐  NO ☐ |
| | Patient is concerned regarding changes in hobbies /leisure activities: | YES ☐  NO ☐ |
| | _____<br>_____<br>_____ | |

| **Registered nurse's signature** | **Grade** | **Date** | **Time** |
|---|---|---|---|
| **Student nurse's signature** | | | |

# Appendix 2 Fluid Balance Chart

**Daily Fluid Balance Chart**

Name: _____

Hospital Number: _____

D. O. B.: _____

Date: _____

| Time | Intake ||||| Output |||||
|---|---|---|---|---|---|---|---|---|---|---|
|  | Oral | NG/PEG | IV Fluid | IV Fluid | Cum Total | Urine | NG/Gastric | DRAIN | STOMA/BOWEL | Cum Total |
| 0800 | | | | | | | | | | |
| 0900 | | | | | | | | | | |
| 1000 | | | | | | | | | | |
| 1100 | | | | | | | | | | |
| 1200 | | | | | | | | | | |
| 1300 | | | | | | | | | | |
| 1400 | | | | | | | | | | |
| 1500 | | | | | | | | | | |
| 1600 | | | | | | | | | | |
| 1700 | | | | | | | | | | |
| 1800 | | | | | | | | | | |
| 1900 | | | | | | | | | | |
| 2000 | | | | | | | | | | |
| 2100 | | | | | | | | | | |
| 2200 | | | | | | | | | | |
| 2300 | | | | | | | | | | |
| 2400 | | | | | | | | | | |
| 0100 | | | | | | | | | | |
| 0200 | | | | | | | | | | |
| 0300 | | | | | | | | | | |
| 0400 | | | | | | | | | | |
| 0500 | | | | | | | | | | |
| 0600 | | | | | | | | | | |
| 0700 | | | | | | | | | | |
| Total: | | | | | | | | | | |

Total Intake: _____ mls

Total Output: _____ mls

Balance: _____ mls        pos/neg

Container Volumes:

Mug/beaker – 200mls

Cup – 150mls  Small glass – 150 mls

Soup bowl – 180mls

# Appendix 3 INEWS Chart

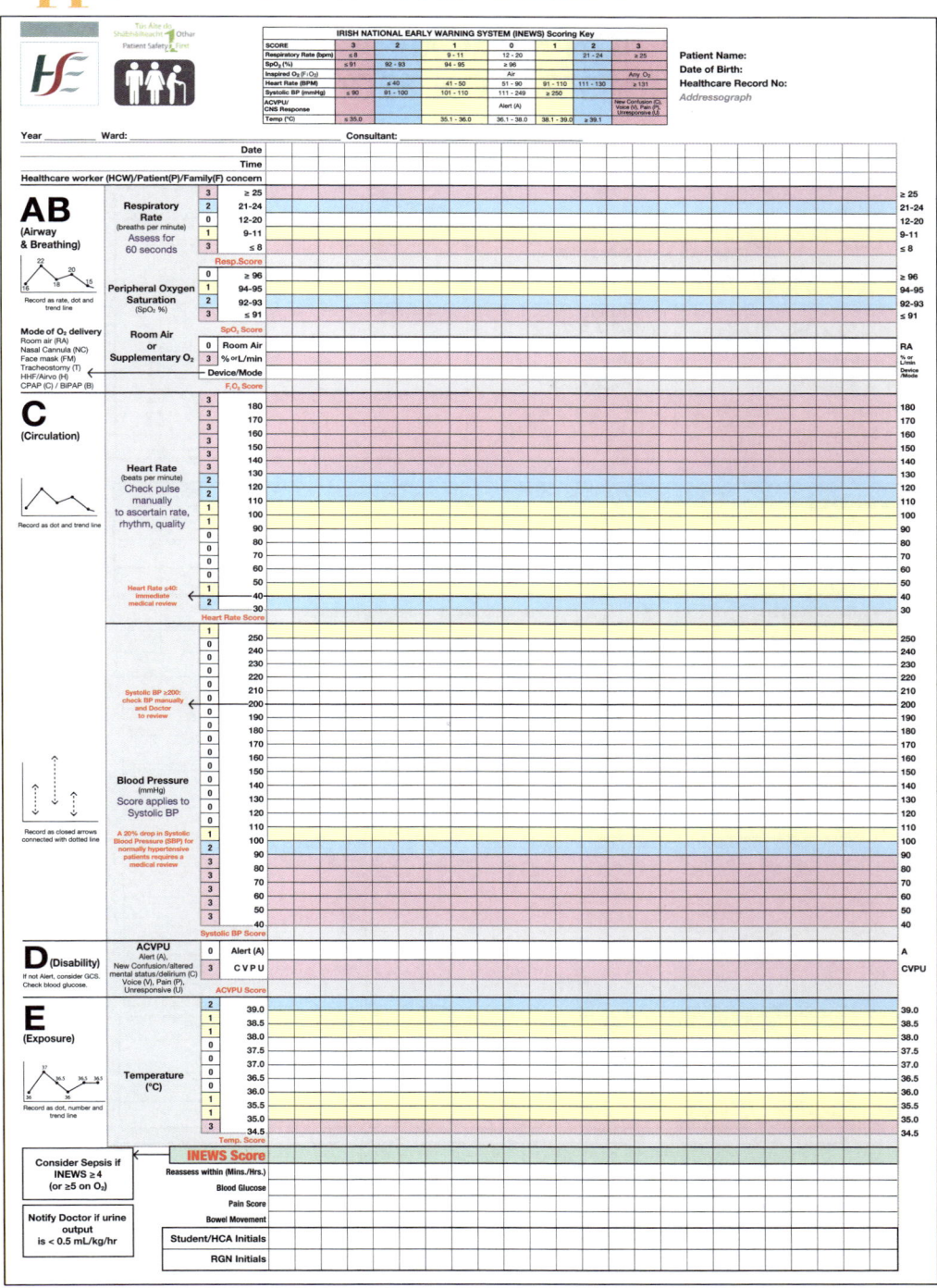

**IRISH NATIONAL EARLY WARNING SYSTEM (INEWS) Scoring Key**

| SCORE | 3 | 2 | 1 | 0 | 1 | 2 | 3 |
|---|---|---|---|---|---|---|---|
| Respiratory Rate (bpm) | ≤ 8 | | 9 - 11 | 12 - 20 | | 21 - 24 | ≥ 25 |
| SpO₂ (%) | ≤ 91 | 92 - 93 | 94 - 95 | ≥ 96 | | | |
| Inspired O₂ (F₁O₂) | | | | Air | | | Any O₂ |
| Heart Rate (BPM) | ≤ 40 | | 41 - 50 | 51 - 90 | 91 - 110 | 111 - 130 | ≥ 131 |
| Systolic BP (mmHg) | ≤ 90 | 91 - 100 | 101 - 110 | 111 - 249 | ≥ 250 | | |
| ACVPU/ CNS Response | | | | Alert (A) | | | New Confusion (C), Voice (V), Pain (P), Unresponsive (U) |
| Temp (°C) | ≤ 35.0 | | 35.1 - 36.0 | 36.1 - 38.0 | 38.1 - 39.0 | ≥ 39.1 | |

Patient Name:
Date of Birth:
Healthcare Record No:
*Addressograph*

Year _____ Ward: _____ Consultant: _____

Date / Time / Healthcare worker (HCW)/Patient(P)/Family(F) concern

**AB** (Airway & Breathing)
Record as rate, dot and trend line
Mode of O₂ delivery: Room air (RA), Nasal Cannula (NC), Face mask (FM), Tracheostomy (T), HHF/Airvo (H), CPAP (C) / BiPAP (B)

Respiratory Rate (breaths per minute) Assess for 60 seconds:
| Score | bpm |
|---|---|
| 3 | ≥ 25 |
| 2 | 21-24 |
| 0 | 12-20 |
| 1 | 9-11 |
| 3 | ≤ 8 |

Peripheral Oxygen Saturation (SpO₂ %):
| Score | % |
|---|---|
| 0 | ≥ 96 |
| 1 | 94-95 |
| 2 | 92-93 |
| 3 | ≤ 91 |

Room Air or Supplementary O₂:
| Score | |
|---|---|
| 0 | Room Air |
| 3 | % or L/min |
| | Device/Mode |

**C** (Circulation)
Record as dot and trend line

Heart Rate (beats per minute) Check pulse manually to ascertain rate, rhythm, quality:
Scores: 3/180, 3/170, 3/160, 3/150, 3/140, 2/130, 2/120, 1/110, 1/100, 0/90, 0/80, 0/70, 0/60, 0/50, 1/40, 2/30
Heart Rate ≤40: immediate medical review

Blood Pressure (mmHg) Score applies to Systolic BP. Record as closed arrows connected with dotted line. Systolic BP ≥200: check BP manually and Doctor to review. A 20% drop in Systolic Blood Pressure (SBP) for normally hypertensive patients requires a medical review.
Scores: 1/250, 0/240, 0/230, 0/220, 0/210, 0/200, 0/190, 0/180, 0/170, 0/160, 0/150, 0/140, 0/130, 0/120, 0/110, 1/100, 2/90, 3/80, 3/70, 3/60, 3/50, 3/40

**D** (Disability)
If not Alert, consider GCS. Check blood glucose.
ACVPU: Alert (A), New Confusion/altered mental status/delirium (C), Voice (V), Pain (P), Unresponsive (U)
| Score | |
|---|---|
| 0 | Alert (A) |
| 3 | CVPU |

**E** (Exposure)
Record as dot, number and trend line

Temperature (°C):
| Score | °C |
|---|---|
| 2 | 39.0 |
| 1 | 38.5 |
| 1 | 38.0 |
| 0 | 37.5 |
| 0 | 37.0 |
| 0 | 36.5 |
| 0 | 36.0 |
| 1 | 35.5 |
| 1 | 35.0 |
| 3 | 34.5 |

**INEWS Score**
Reassess within (Mins./Hrs.)
Blood Glucose
Pain Score
Bowel Movement
Student/HCA Initials
RGN Initials

Consider Sepsis if INEWS ≥ 4 (or ≥5 on O₂)

Notify Doctor if urine output is < 0.5 mL/kg/hr

*Source:* https://assets.gov.ie/87927/38dfaa00-05c7-4c37-9fc5-4814e0c1b38b.pdf

# Appendix 4 Medication Chart

## MEDICATION PRESCRIPTION AND ADMINISTRATION RECORD

Please use a **BLACK BALLPOINT** pen when writing on this prescription record

Affix addressograph here

| | |
|---|---|
| **PATIENT NAME** | |
| **ADDRESS** | Resident at Capola Home, Ridgewood, Kildare. |
| **DATE OF BIRTH** | 31/08/1946 |
| **HOSPITAL NUMBER** | 07973308 |
| **PATIENT GENDER** | Female |
| **ADMISSION DATE** | 01/06/2015 |
| **HEIGHT** | 5 ft 2 in |
| **ADMISSION WEIGHT (Kg)** | 70 kg |
| **NEW WT.** | 70 kg DATE 01/06/2015 |
| **NEW WT.** | 70 kg DATE 05/06/2015 |

| | |
|---|---|
| **CONSULTANT DOCTOR IN CHARGE** | Dr Paul Smith |
| **MEDICAL REG. NO** | 0000126 |
| **WARD** | Capola Nursing Home |

**OTHER MEDICATION RECORDS IN USE** (please tick)
- INSULIN ☐   TPN ☐
- CHEMOTHERAPY ☐   NUTRITION ☐
- BLOOD PRODUCTS ☐   PCA ☐
- EPIDURAL ☐   HAEMODIALYSIS ☐
- OTHER ☐ ____

### UNDERLYING CONDITIONS AFFECTING PRESCRIBING (please tick appropriate box initial and date)

| Renal Impairment | Hepatic Impairment | Overweight / Underweight | Swallowing Difficulties | Pregnancy | Breastfeeding | Other (please specify) |
|---|---|---|---|---|---|---|
| Initial: | Initial: | Initial: | Initial: | Initial: | Initial: | Initial: |
| Date: | Date: | Date: | Date: | Date: | Date: | Date: |

Is the patient a smoker?   Yes ☐   No ☑   If yes, please consider referral for smoking cessation

**Oral Medication in Surgical Pre Operative Patients**
Patients who are "nill-by-mouth", awaiting surgery **MUST** receive their usual oral medication (accept oral hypoglycaemics) unless the prescription has been cancelled.

### ALLERGIES, SENSITIVITIES OR CONTRAINDICTIONS
Nurses cannot administer any medications unless this is completed and signed by a prescriber or a pharmacist.

The patient has no known allergies ☐   Signature and bleep ____   Date ____

| Name of Drug | Type of Allergy | State if drug to be used with caution or contraindicated | Signature, bleep and date |
|---|---|---|---|
| | | | |
| | | | |
| | | | |
| | | | |
| | | | |
| | | | |

### MEDICINES RECONCILIATION ON ADMISSION

Admission Time: 9.00 am   Date: 01/06/2015
Medication Reconciled at: 2.00 pm   (Date) 01/06/2015
SOURCE OF INFORMATION   Medical Notes ☑   GP ☑   Patient ☑   Pharmacist ☑

### REGULAR PRESCRIPTIONS FOR MEDICINES TO BE ADMINISTERED DURING REGULAR MEDICAL ROUNDS

| PRESCRIPTION | DOSE | DATE → | | | | | | |
|---|---|---|---|---|---|---|---|---|
| DRUG (APPROVED NAME) Lanzoprazole | | 0800 | | | | | | |
| | | 1000 | | | | | | |
| FREQUENCY Daily   ROUTE   START DATE 01/06/2015   REVIEW DATE 4 weeks | | 1200 | | | | | | |
| | | 1400 | | | | | | |
| | | 1600 | | | | | | |
| PRESCRIBER'S SIGNATURE   STOP DATE | | 1800 | | | | | | |
| PHARMACIST | | 2000 | | | | | | |
| | | 2200 | | | | | | |

# Index

abbreviations, 197
activities of daily living, 39–44, 49, 72, 82
   factors which influence, 43
acute hospitals, 14, 25, 27, 62, 192
Advanced Nurse Practitioner (ANP), 13, 18, 192, 197
advocacy, 56, 61–62, 206
airborne precautions see transmission-based precautions, 134
alcohol hand rub 114
   technique 114
An Bord Altranais, see NMBI, 8, 10, 13
anatomy, 75–78
   ligaments, 78
   nerves, 78
   skeletal muscles, 77
   spine, 75
   tendons, 77
antibiotics, 107, 129–132
apnoea, see respiration, 159
autonomy, also see ethics, 169–171, 193
   negative, 169
   positive, 169

Bachelor of Science (BSc) Honours Nursing, 16
bacteria, 107, 119, 126, 128–132
beneficence, see ethics, 169, 170, 171
biomechanics, 72, 73, 77, 78–79
   centre of gravity, 78–79
blood pressure, 138, 147, 155, 161–165, 166
   diastolic pressure, 162
   factors affecting, 163
   hypotension, 162, 163
   hypertension, 162
   procedure for taking, 164
   recording, 165
   systolic pressure, 162
blood/bodily secretions, see modes of transmission, 116
blood-borne viruses, 125–127
   Hepatitis B, 126
   Hepatitis C, 126
   HIV/AIDS, 126
body temperature, 137, 138, 147–154
   hypothermia, 89, 149, 197
   hyperthermia, 197
   measuring and recording, 148–154, 197
bradycardia, see pulse, 155, 197
bradypnoea, see respiration, 159

buccal (BC), 180
burns, 130, 138

cancer care, 29–30
Catholic nuns, 4
   Daughters of Charity, 4
   Sisters of Mercy, 2, 5
Central Midwives Board, 5
chain of infection, 104, 110–111
   infectious agent, 110
   means of transmission, 110
   portal of entry, 110
   portal of exit, 110
   reservoir, 110
   susceptible host, 111
charts, see medical/medication charts, 28, 133, 134, 135
clinical nurse specialist (CNS), 13, 18
clostridium difficile, see HCAIs, 128–129
code of ethics for nurses, 171–173
Code of Practice for Healthcare Records Management, 197
Code of Professional Conduct and Ethics, 172–173, 192, 195
colonisation, 129
Commission on Nursing, 11–15, 18, 19
communication, 27, 52, 132,
   in ethics, 169, 171
   in the lifespan continuum, 42
   in nursing, 57, 68, 195
   in people moving/handling, 90, 91,
   in relationships with patients, 60–62
community care, 18, 25, 30
confidentiality, see ethics, 35, 50, 59, 69, 133, 134, 136, 168–172
consent, see ethics, 168, 169, 171
contaminated linen, see linen and laundry, 121–123
contraindication, see medication administration, 178
COVID-19, 105
CPE/CRE, see bacteria, 132
Crimean War, 5, 7
cross-infection, see micro-organisms, 108–110, 111, 125, 150

decontamination of equipment, 112, 118–119, 133, 135, 136
dehydration, 128–129, 163, 183
Department of Health, 22–24, 175
diarrhoea, 105, 127, 128, 131, 138, 142

diastolic (see blood pressure), 162–165
direct transmission, see modes of transmission, 109
EU directives, 18, 20, 191
Director of Nursing (DON), 18
disinfection, 118, 119, 133, 135, 136
diuretics, 138
droplet precautions, see transmission-based precautions, 132, 135–136
drugs, see medication management, 176–188
  administration of, 179–196
  controlled drugs, 186–187
  legislation, 177
  medication errors, 188
  recording and documentation, 188
dyspnoea, see respiration, 159

Early Warning system (EWS), 147, 166–167
economic recession, 14
empathic behaviour examples, 139, 140, 141, 153, 157, 159, 161
empathy, 36, 56–62, 171
employee duties, see people moving and handling, 78–79
employer duties, see people moving and handling, 78
Enlightenment, the, 5
ethics, 168–173, 178, 192, 194
  autonomy, 169
  beneficence, 170
  confidentiality, 170
  consent, 171
  non-maleficence, 170
European Union, 9
evidence-based practice, 33–34

faecal-oral transmission, see modes of transmission, 110
Fitness to Practice Committee, 10, 19
Five Moments for Hand Hygiene, 112
Florence Nightingale, 5–7
fluid balance
  calculating the balance, 142
  fluid balance chart, 137, 140–146, 218
  fluid balance practice, 143–146
  measuring and recording, 140–147
fluid overload, 139
fungal infections, 181
fungi, see micro-organisms, 106, 108

general nursing, 13, 15, 16, 17
General Nursing Council, 8
Gibbs' reflective cycle, 63–67

hand hygiene, 111–114, 115, 118
HCAIs (healthcare-associated infection), 125, 127–132
Health Act 2004, 24

Health and Safety Authority (HSA), 73, 74, 75
Health Information and Quality Authority (HIQA), 31–32, 176, 178
  inspections, 32
Health Service Executive (HSE), 24–25, 197
  medication administration, 178, 188
  nurses in, 30–31
  specialist cancer care, 29–30
  tertiary Care, 30
Health, Department of, 22–24, 175
Hepatitis B, see blood-borne viruses, 125–126
Hepatitis C, see blood-borne viruses, 126–126
HIV and AIDS, see blood-borne viruses, 126–127
hoists, 72, 88–89, 90, 99
holistic care, 33, 37, 178
hypertension, see blood pressure, 162–163
hyperthermia/pyrexia, 149, 197
hypotension, see blood pressure, 162–163

indication, see medication administration, 178
indirect transmission, see cross-infection, 109
industrial action, 13, 62
infection prevention and control, 104–123
infectious agent, Chain of Infection, 110–111, 132
infusions, 142, 182–184
injections, 76, 182–184
intellectual disability nursing, 17
interpersonal skills, see communication, 52, 57–58, 60, 62
intervertebral discs, see Anatomy, 76
intramuscular injection (IM), 183
intravenous infusion, 184
intravenous injection (IV), 183
Irish Medicines Board Act (IMB), 177
Irish Medicines Board (Miscellaneous Provisions) Act (2006), 177
Irish Nurses' Organisation, 13

Kant, Immanuel, 169

Labour Court, 12, 13, 15
lifting guidelines, 80–82
ligaments, see anatomy, 75, 76, 78
linen and laundry, 112, 121–123

MDA (Misuse of Drugs Act), 177, 186–187
means of transmission, see chain of infection, 110–111
medical charts, 28
medication chart, 186, 188, 220

# INDEX

medication management, 173, 176–188
  administrating medication, 178–184
  controlled drugs, 186–187
  legislation, 177
  medication errors, 188
  recording and documentation, 188
  safety, 184–186
Medicinal Products Regulations 2003, 187
microbiology, 106
micro-organisms, 106–108, 112, 116, 117, 118, 119
Midwives Act, 19, 172
Mill, John Stuart, 169
Misuse of Drugs Acts (MDA), 177, 186–187
modes of transmission, 109–110
  blood and bodily secretions, 110
  direct, 109
  droplet/airborne transmission, 109
  faecal-oral transmission, 110
  indirect, 109
  skin/Direct Contact, 109
models of nursing, 37–48
  Benner, 37
  Neuman, 37
  Orem, 38
  Roper, Logan and Tierney, 39–44

nasal cavity, 182
nasal secretions, 109
needlestick injuries, 112, 120–121
nerves, see anatomy, 75, 76, 77, 78
Nightingale, Florence, 5–7
NMBI, 9, 16–19, 61, 68, 174, 178, 191, 193
non-maleficence, see ethics, 168, 169, 170–171
non-risk waste, 119
Norovirus, see HCAIs, 107, 128, 130–131
nurse prescriber, 17
Nurses Act 1950, 8, 20
Nurses Act 1961, 20
Nurses Act 1985, 10, 13, 19, 20
Nurses and Midwives Act 2011, 19, 20, 172
Nurses Registration Act 1919, 8
Nursing and Midwifery Board of Ireland (NMBI), 9, 16–19, 61, 68, 174, 178, 191, 193
Nursing Education Forum, 12
nursing process, 33, 48–55, 170
nursing unions, 12, 13
nursing values, 34–36

objective data, see nursing process, 50
observations, 68, 69, 140
  Early Warning System (EWS), 166–167
  physiological observations, 147–167
one-arm loads, see safe lifting guidelines, 81
opthalmic, 182
oral administration (PO), 179–180

Orem's self-care model, see nursing models, 38
otic administration, 182

pain medication, 76
parasites, 106, 108
partnership, see person-centred care, 35, 40, 45, 52, 58, 141
patient transfer techniques, 83
people moving and handling, 82
  communication, 91
  manual handling, 72–75, 86
  principles, 82
  risk assessment, 73, 83–90
  safe lifting guidelines, 80–82
  techniques, 83, 91–92, 93–103
  TILE, 84–90
personal protective equipment (PPE), 80, 106, 115–117
person-centred care, 30, 35, 58, 105
pharmacology, 179
physiological observations, 147–167
  blood pressure, 161–165
  body temperature, 148–154
  pulse, 155–157
  respiration, 158–161
patient care, 68, 191
  manual handling, 76, 84
  nursing process, 49
polypharmacy, 179
portal of entry, see chain of infection, 110, 111
portal of exit, see chain of infection, 110, 111
positive self-image, 36, 59
post-registration programmes, 16
primary care, 25, 26–27, 28, 38
privacy and dignity, 35, 58, 171
  examples in practice, 141, 153, 157, 161, 165
professional socialisation, see scope of practice, 190
protective isolation, 123
psychiatric nursing, 16, 17
pulmonary arteries, veins, 161
pulmonary disease, 156, 158
pulmonary drug preparation, 181
pulse, 147, 155–157
  measuring, recording the pulse, 156–157
pulse oximetry, 160–161
pulse rate, 157
  brachial pulse, 156
  bradycardia, 155, 197
  carotid pulse, 156
  tachycardia, 155

raising a client, see people moving and handling techniques, 100–103

223

record-keeping, 68–70, 186
  rules, 69
recording clinical practice, 69–70
recruitment embargo, 14
rectal (PR), 181
reflective practice, 56, 63–67, 191
  reflection in-action, 63
  reflection on-action, 63
relationships, 39, 60–61, 173, 195
  therapeutic, 52, 60–62, 140, 141, 170
reporting, 68–70
repositioning a client, *see* people moving and handling techniques, 102–103
reservoir, *see* chain of infection, 110–111
respect, 35, 58, 83, 87, 93, 169–173
respiration, 158–161
  abnormalities, 159
  breathing assessment, 158
respiratory precautions, 117–118
risk assessment, 73, 83–90, 132,
risk waste, 119
rolling a client, *see* people moving and handling techniques, 95–97
  activities of daily living, 39–40
  dependence/independence continuum, 41–42
  factors influencing, 43–44, 47
  individuality in living, 44
  lifespan, 41
  model of living, 39–48
  model of nursing, 44–46
  Roper, N., Logan, W. and Tierney, A. 39–48, 215–217

safe lifting guidelines, 80–82
safe management of waste, 119–123
Safety, Health and Welfare at Work (General Application) 2007 Regulations, 87, 90
Saint Catherine of Siena, 4
saturation levels, 160–161
scope of nursing and midwifery practice, 61, 193–195
Scope of Nursing and Midwifery Practice Framework 2015, 61
scope of practice, 190–195
  decision making chart, 194
  professional socialisation, 190
secondary care, 27–28
sepsis, 131, 149, 167
sharps, safe disposal of, 120–121
sit to stand, *see* people moving and handling techniques, 93–95
skeletal muscles, *see* anatomy, 75, 77
skin/direct contact, *see* modes of transmission, 109
Sláintecare, 23, 25
slide sheets, *see* people moving and handling techniques 97–99

soiled linen, *see* linen and laundry, 121, 122–123
spine, *see* anatomy, 75, 76–77
St. Vincent de Paul, 4
standard precautions, 104, 111–123, 125, 126, 132–135
staphylococcus aureus (Staph.), 128, 129–130
sterilisation, 118, 119
strike action, 12, 15
subcutaneous infusion, 183
subcutaneous injection (SC), 183
subjective data, *see* nursing process, 50, 70
sublingual (SL), 180
supernumerary, 11
susceptible host, *see* chain of infection, 111
sweating/fever, 138
systolic blood pressure, 162, 164

tachycardia, 155, 197
tachypnoea, *see* respiration, 159
temperature (body), 40, 42, 137, 138, 147
  measuring and recording, 148–151
  methods of measuring, 151–154
tendons, *see* anatomy, 75, 76, 77
tertiary care, 26, 29–31
thermometers, 150–151
  digital, 150
  disposable, 150
  tympanic, 150
TILE, 84–90
training schools, 6, 7
transdermal (TD), 180
transmission-based precautions, 125, 132–136
two-person lift, *see* people moving and handling techniques, 81

urination, 138

vaginal (PV), 181
viruses, 105, 106–107, 119, 125, 126
vital signs, 147–165
vomiting, 127, 131, 139, 143–146
VRE, *see* bacteria, 131–132

World Health Organization, 112